BEHIND THE MASK

How the World Survived SARS

The First Epidemic of the 21st Century

by Tim Brookes

with Omar A. Khan, MD, MHS
Technical Consultant

American Public Health Association

American Public Health Association
800 I Street, NW
Washington, DC 20001–3710
www.apha.org

Cover photographs courtesy of the Information Services Department of the Hong Kong SAR Government, except inset center and right photographs courtesy of the CDC Public Health Image Library. Used with permission.

Georges C. Benjamin, MD, FACP
Executive Director

Printed and bound in the United States of America
Set In: Janson Text
Interior Design and Typesetting: Terry Anderson
Cover Design: Michele Pryor
Printing and Binding by Cadmus Professional Communications

ISBN 0-87553-046-X
2M 10/04

Table of Contents

1. Red Herrings, Red Flags 1

2. Rumors and Remedies 11

3. GOARN 21

4. Too Many Viruses 27

5. Global Warning, Global Alarm 33

6. At the Metropole 39

7. The Outbreak Spreads 47

8. Where the Hell Is This Guy? 57

9. In the Hospitals 73

10. The Worst Days: A Near Miss 95

11. Racing the Virus 101

12. One Deep: A Case Study in Public Health in Toronto 121

13. Amoy Gardens 141

14. Removing the Handle 149

15. Singapore: A Case Study in Quarantine 161

16. People Would Move Away: SARS and Stigma 185

17. Dire Straits: China and Taiwan 193

18. It Wasn't Magic Any More 213

19. Aftershocks 223

20. Learning from SARS 233

APPENDICES:

Afterword: Georges C. Benjamin, MD, FACP 235

Dialogue: WHO's David Heymann and Guenael Rodier 237

Timeline: SARS 243

Annotated Bibliography 247

About the Author 252

Index 253

Acknowledgements

Dozens of people gave significant amounts of their time and attention, often at very short notice, to help with this book. Many of them also took the professional risk of being candid about a situation that was novel, confusing, arduous and even out of control. In particular I'd like to thank the following:

At the World Health Organization in Geneva: Dick Thompson, Mike Ryan, Angela Merianos, Guenael Rodier, Klaus Stohr, Mary Kay Kindhauser, Ellah Frodeman, Siobhan Landecy, Julie Symons, Denise Werker, Annette Chanel, and especially Garry Smyth.

In Hong Kong: Kwok-Yung Yuen, Mary Waye, Paul Tam, Lo Su Vui, Andrew Yip, Fred Leung, Lily Chiu, David Hui, Chan Kwok Hung, Karen Richardson, Daisy CY Lo, Alan Chan, Raymond HY Li.

In China: Tan Yue-Qiu, Zhongan Zhu. In Taiwan: Pei-Jer Chen, Julian Wu. In England: David Fidler. At the WHO around the world: Pascale Brudon, Henk Bekedam, Bob Dietz, Nguyen Thuc Anh.

In Toronto: Peter Macintyre, Barbara Switzer, Jane Speakman, Barbara Yaffe, Rita Shahin, Tanya Kumar, Karietha Cooke, Mark Bartlett, Carola Ostach, Tom Marjanovich, Les Shulman, Corinne Shopman and especially Anna Miranda, Geri Nephew and Bonnie Henry.

In the United States: John Thanassi, Ellen Meyer, Anne Schuchat, Jon Liden, Maybelis Fernandez, Dr. James Hughes, and Richard Lowe.

This book would never have got off the ground without the invaluable assistance from Jen-Fu Chiu, David Heymann, my indefatigable friend and colleague Omar Khan and my wife Barbara.

To all those who struggled
to understand and contain SARS,
to those who died trying,
and to their families.

Chapter 1.

Red Herrings, Red Flags

Nobody knows that an epidemic is starting. By definition, an epidemic is already under way; it already has a disturbing and dangerous momentum.

It's even harder to know that an epidemic of an entirely new infectious disease has begun. Everything is confusion and turmoil. Everyone makes mistakes.

This was especially true of SARS, given that its greatest and most lethal trick was its ability to disguise itself, to mask itself behind the symptoms of other diseases.

The best way to understand the beginning of the SARS epidemic, then, is to go back to a mistake, a series of mistakes, many of which actually had nothing to do with what would come to be identified as the new SARS coronavirus, but the mistakes themselves would dictate how the epidemic was perceived and understood, or misunderstood. We need to go back to January 2, 2003, when the Hong Kong government officially reopened the border between Hong Kong and mainland China to chickens.

This was generally seen in Hong Kong as good news. The Chinese New Year was only six weeks away, and chicken (traditionally selected live, then killed and eaten fresh) is always a staple in Chinese home and restaurant cooking during the several days of New Year celebrations. Many Hong Kong and mainland residents use chickens to worship Buddha and their ancestors during festivals, so a chicken shortage would have been a major inconvenience.

One person who was less than wholeheartedly enthusiastic about the development was Dr. Frederick C. Leung, a professor in the Department of Zoology of the University of Hong Kong.

Fred Leung looks like what he is: a scientist who works with farmers. A strongly built man of medium height, open shirt, jeans, and sneakers, he speaks his mind with unusual freedom for someone who is also the dean of the faculty of science of a major university. He spent fifteen years in the U.S., getting his Ph.D. from the University of California and then working as a specialist in agricultural pathogens, and he was the specialist who was contacted in 1996 when, in farms all around the Pearl River Delta, chickens began dying.

The Pearl River Delta is historically one of the most important areas of China. The Pearl River flows roughly southeast through the South China province of Guangdong, past the major cities of Shenzhen, Zhongshan, Foshan, and the provincial capital Guangzhou, formerly known in the West as Canton, before passing between the two island-cities of Hong Kong and Macau, set on each side of it like the twin pillars of Western imperial history in the Orient, and emptying into the China Sea.

It was precisely because the Pearl River was such a major waterway and Hong Kong such a strategically perfect port that the British kept it as a colony long after relinquishing any substantial presence in mainland China. Any goods that China wished to export must now pass through Hong Kong and pay tariffs; conversely, Hong Kong became a major marketplace for Western goods to be sold to people coming from the Western Pacific region in general and mainland China in particular. Even after the British lease on Hong Kong expired in 1997 and the island-city became the Hong Kong Special Administrative Region (SAR), a province of China, Hong Kong retained its Janus-like status in the region, looking both into China and out to the world. As travel restrictions between China and Hong Kong were relaxed and tourists from the heartland began flooding into the new province, this curious ambidextrous stance became still more pronounced.

The group of 237 islands that makes up Hong Kong is only a small part of the Delta, which put Fred Leung in an almost unique vantage position: from 1996 onward, in working with chicken and pig farmers around the Delta, he saw firsthand what was happening in agriculture on both sides of the border. This panorama involved nothing less than being able to see into the future of infectious disease.

At the time, though, it wasn't clear how important that view was, or would turn out to be. Leung suspected that the culprit in the chicken deaths was IBDV—Infectious Bursal Disease Virus, a highly virulent pathogen with a mortality rate of 80-90%. He obtained a sample in early 1997, sequenced it, and sure enough it was IBDV.

"Coincidentally, in early 1997, when we were collecting samples around the Pearl River Delta on other projects, we heard chicken farmers saying, 'This year is really bad. A lot of birds are dying.'"

That in itself was a disturbing sign. Viruses have a peculiar relationship to their hosts: a virus is such a rudimentary entity—barely more than a shell containing some strands of genetic material—that on its own it can barely be said to be alive. It is unable to reproduce on its own, needing instead to attach itself to a cell in a host creature of some kind, dissolve a tiny hole in the cell wall, and send in some of its own genetic strands. These strands find the nucleus of the cell, and insert themselves into the process by which a cell reproduces itself. The infected cell, instead (or in addition to) making copies of itself, makes copies of the virus: millions of them; so many, in fact, that they can fill the cell, burst it open and spill out, each one ready to dock onto another cell and repeat the process.

Over time, a virus develops strategies that enable it to survive in a host, sometimes to mutual benefit. Each of us has substantial numbers of viruses in our bodies at any given time, not doing us any appreciable harm. But every time a virus reproduces, genetic variations occur. This happens in any form of reproduction apart from cloning, but in more complex organisms such as humans, each cell has a mechanism for checking that the DNA has reproduced itself accurately, and an allied mechanism for repairing any sections of DNA that have errors in them. Viruses, reduced to the essential components, lack both these mechanisms, so they change and evolve rapidly.

Most of these genetic variations, also called mutations, make no apparent difference because they take place in the long stretches of DNA that have no function that we can discern (geneticists call it "garbage DNA"). Some mutations, however, take place in a crucial section of DNA, dramatically altering its activities in some way that affects its relationship with the host. From an evolutionary point of view, it is not in the virus's interest to kill the host: a virus is unable to reproduce in a dead host, and will likely itself die. So when a host dies of a viral infection, something radical has happened to a virus—it has become a loose cannon of sorts.

Something like this had happened to a chicken virus, and it was Fred Leung's job to find out what.

"Well, you know that inside China, information is not usually readily available," he explained in his lab, surrounded by genetics books and photos of sick farmyard animals. “The central government claims that they have no foot-and-mouth disease, and no avian influenza—it’s hard to go against what the government has said. But we noticed a lot of unconfirmed reports of chickens dying. At first we thought it was just IBDV, but from what the farmers were saying and from the fact that ducks and geese [were dying] made us wonder if it might be a new virus.”

It was indeed a new virus: H5N1, the Avian Influenza (AI) or bird flu virus, which the Hong Kong University Department of Microbiology isolated, identified, and described for the scientific literature. And that, everyone thought, was that. After all, this was only zoology, a discipline that in a university science hierarchy is often seen a rung below the “purer” sciences such as physics, genetics or microbiology, and is thus taken less seriously. Many major human diseases are zoonotic—that is, they originate in animals—but in the hierarchy of disciplines in modern medicine, zoology ranks only slightly above metalwork shop and home economics.

H5N1 might have remained merely a nuisance virus like IBDV: dangerous to fowl and costly to farmers but irrelevant to most others. By chance, however, something happened that could only occur in a farming community.

Humans, pigs, and chickens have a fair number of biological similarities, and one of them is that all three can get colds and flu. In other words, all three can host viruses causing the common cold, as well as influenza viruses, though how each of the three reacts to each virus varies considerably. In an agricultural setting, the three species pass germs back and forth surprisingly often: pigs sneeze, chickens cough, and the farmer is in close proximity with both, doing his own share of coughing and sneezing. Viruses are also shed in large quantities in feces, and nobody ever claimed that a farmer’s life was a sanitary one.

Sometime in 1996 or 1997, the avian influenza virus that by now was fairly widespread in the Pearl River Delta mutated again, but in a different way: somehow, a bird virus and a human virus both infected the same cell, possibly in a pig, and the pig’s cell began to produce offspring viruses that were genetically a combination of both bird and human virus. As a bird virus, it was not genetically adapted to survive and flourish in a human host, but, to oversimplify somewhat, this accidental grafting gave it just enough human DNA to jump the species gap.

In point of fact, this probably happened many, many times: for a single virus to mutate and start an epidemic is the stuff of science fiction. In early summer of 1997, one of these viruses found a human host: a three-year-old boy who was admitted to Hong Kong's Queen Elizabeth Hospital in early May. His immune system had never seen anything like the H5N1 virus—quite possibly, no human being's immune system ever had—and could not recognize it as a potential danger. The virus multiplied unchecked, making hundreds of thousands of copies of itself in the first day alone. In less than two weeks the boy died of a massive viral invasion causing a bewildering array of symptoms: pneumonia, acute respiratory distress, Reye's syndrome (liver and brain damage), and multiple organ system failures.

At the time, Leung explained, the boy's death was a mystery. "It was really, really nasty, but there was no so-called cause of death." Pathology sent a sample to Microbiology, who were unable to diagnose it, though they recognized that it was flu-like in nature. The sample was sent on, not to Leung's lab but to the U.S. Centers for Disease Control and Prevention (CDC) in Atlanta, who sequenced it and found it to be "avian-like influenza," or a virus similar to H5N1. This was regarded as a curiosity but little more, according to Leung. Science wrote what he called "a very short blip" about it noting that this was the first time an avian gene sequence had been found in a human virus. "Then the whole thing died down."

In October 1997, the chicken farmers in mainland China and Hong Kong began reporting that chickens were dying again, and in November the outbreak began infecting humans. Eighteen people were infected in Hong Kong, of whom six died: a shocking rate of lethality on par with smallpox, albeit in a small number of people.

Hong Kong, China, and the world were saved from a terrifying epidemic by a vital fact about viruses and how they evolve. It takes one major genetic accident for an animal virus to be able to survive and multiply in a human. It takes another different genetic accident, or even a series of accidents, for that virus to be able to become a human virus, capable of being transmitted from one human to another. The notorious "Spanish" Flu pandemic of 1918-1919 (which originated not in Spain, but likely in the US) probably crossed back and forth several times between humans, birds, and pigs before it acquired its ultimate virulence.

In Hong Kong in late 1997, that series of viral developments had not yet taken place. Humans could catch the virus only from fowl, and with this in mind, the Hong Kong government decided to slaughter every chicken in Hong Kong. The border to mainland China was closed to live chickens, nearly one and a half million chickens in the Hong Kong Special Administrative Region were killed, the outbreak was stopped, and the Hong Kong government was praised for its painful but necessary drastic action.

Leung argued against the slaughter, though nobody in authority listened to him. "Personally, I was against killing all the chickens. Killing infected chickens, yes. I also agree with killing chickens that have come into contact with infected chickens. That's also the WHO [World Health Organization] guideline. Killing all the chickens in a city, or a province, or a country—to me, that's irrational, especially with a deadly virus. With a deadly virus, all you have to do is [contain] it. The infected will die; whoever is still alive didn't contract the virus. I understand why they did it, but the decision was political and economic. It wasn't hazard-based."

It was also shortsighted, in three crucial respects. First, killing the chickens didn't kill the virus. As we now know, avian influenza went underground. With little effective monitoring, in five years it had spread throughout Southeast Asia and had reached North America. For this reason, Leung is not a fan of efforts to eradicate specific diseases. "The virus will evolve, irrespective. You do things to block it, and it will go around them, or over them, or dig underneath, and you still won't be able to stop it. Look at what happened with smallpox. Look at what happened with polio, the two viruses we've managed to 'eradicate': they've turned into bioterrorism agents."

Second, killing all the chickens dealt a very severe blow to Hong Kong chicken farmers ("The industry took a very, very deep hit"), forcing Hong Kong to import still more chickens from the mainland. Agricultural monitoring and certification in Hong Kong take place at levels that, according to Leung, are as scrupulous as those in the West. In mainland China, he suggests, certification is less rigorous.

"We have no way of telling mainland [China] farmers what to do. We can only monitor right at the gates. We can't be self-sufficient; we have to import, so the choice is to import live chickens and live pigs, or killed chickens and killed pigs. If you don't have any confidence in the certification—you can buy a certificate—then live chickens and live pigs are still better than 'meat products.' I'd rather see a live bird or a live pig, so I can make sure they don't have any disease, and then let them in and process them. Then I have some quality control."

Third, the culling of chickens gave the impression that infectious disease could be dealt with in one's own backyard—something that has rarely been true and is often fatally wrong. Infectious diseases, as we are reminded time and time again, do not respect national borders. In addition, by 1997 it had become increasingly clear that (a) with the increase of international travel, disease also traveled more easily, and (b) traditional methods and regulations for quarantine and the interdiction of infection were hopelessly out of date.

But Hong Kong alone could not change the world. It would take a fright of global proportions to change the self-interested mentalities of a hundred countries and the way they dealt with epidemics.

It would come to be called Severe Acute Respiratory Syndrome, or SARS. It would come to be called the first major global epidemic of the twenty-first century, the first epidemic to be spread at the speed of jet aircraft, and the century's first new fatal disease organism.

As things turned out, the chickens were, as every infectious disease specialist with a sense of humor put it, red herrings. But their story overlapped with, and was confused with that of SARS. It introduced the major players in the SARS outbreak: China, Hong Kong, official silence and denial, animals raised for food, a new virus jumping species, a porous international border. The chickens also succeeded SARS, as the next epidemic to follow after SARS was suppressed was avian influenza, now on a global scale. The red herrings were also red flags.

The question of whether avian influenza or SARS would change the way the world deals with emerging infectious diseases, though, is still an open one.

* * *

Officially, killing all the chickens in Hong Kong had contained the spread of avian influenza, but as Leung knew very well, the virus had a natural reservoir—chickens, ducks and geese—all around the Pearl River Delta, and it was only a matter of time before it returned. Between January 1998 and December 1, 2002, there were three outbreaks in Hong Kong, but no new cases of human infection.

In December 2002, though, unofficial reports crossed the border that geese and ducks had been dying on the mainland again. The same reports said that the Chinese government had been suppressing information on the reappearance of the virus. At the same time, avian flu was detected in Penfold Park in the Sha Tin racecourse in Hong

Kong, killing thirty-one ducks, geese and swans, and thirty-eight chickens were found to have died of H5N1, in five live-animal markets. Later, two chicken farms were also found to have been infected, plus the spacious gardens of Kowloon Park.

Paul Chan Kay-sheung, associate professor at the Department of Microbiology at Chinese University and a member of the Hospital Authority's infectious diseases task force, was quoted by newspapers warning that the fowl deaths might be a sign that the virus had mutated. "If it is spreading you would think it might be more virulent and may be quite infectious," he said. "If this is the case, we should step up our monitoring and try to see if any human beings have been in close contact with the birds."

It would have been a miracle if humans had not been in contact with the birds, given that Penfold Park is in the middle of a racecourse that attracts thousands of visitors each weekend and Kowloon Park is in one of the province's busiest tourist areas. The remaining 60 waterfowl at Penfold Park were slaughtered as a precaution, but parrots which the Jockey Club keeps in nearby cages showed no signs of illness and were spared. Horses were said not to be at risk. The Jockey Club said the International Races would go ahead.

And the border between Hong Kong and mainland China was closed to chickens.

But by the beginning of January the danger seemed to have passed. Dr. Yeoh Eng-kiong, the Hong Kong Secretary for Health, said: "What we are seeing now is H5N1, but its internal genotype is slightly different. There is no evidence that this particular strain of bird flu goes into humans." To prevent bird flu from spreading in Hong Kong this time, the local administration decided to disinfect and clean its markets and chicken sales booths over the coming week.

Officials in mainland China were offended by the implication that disease appearing in Hong Kong might have been bred in Guangdong and exported. Any H5 virus found in Hong Kong, said Li Changjiang, the Director of the State Council's Quarantine Office, was homegrown, and all mainland chickens sold in the territory were safe to eat. Yes, he said, there had been cases of bird flu in Guangdong, but the virus had been kept under control.

The border was reopened to chickens. Despite the scare, the chickens fetched almost the same price as the previous year's, and a Guangdong official predicted that his province's chicken exports would soon increase because of the rapidly-approaching Chinese New Year at the end of January.

The first batch of chickens to cross through the border checkpoint numbered about 80,000. Roughly one in four had been given blood tests for the H5N1 virus; all the results were said to be negative.

"We promised," said an official of the Guangdong Provincial Bureau of Foreign Trade and Economic Cooperation, with an air of sanctimonious denial, "to sell only healthy chickens to Hong Kong."

Chapter 2.

Rumors and Remedies

It was a sign of the times, and one of great significance in the field of emerging infectious diseases, that electronic dissemination of information via cell phones and email trumped more traditional methods at stopping the flow. While the Chinese government was still trying to contain information about the strange clusters of fatal illness that were breaking out in the province of Guangdong, the news burst out like a cluster of viruses from their host cell, arriving by phone, email, and pager not only in Hong Kong but in suburban Washington, D.C.

On February 10, Dr. Stephen Cunnion, a consultant in infectious diseases who was formerly with the U.S. Navy, received an alarming email from China. It puzzled him, so he posted an email of his own on ProMED-mail, a list serve run by the International Society for Infectious Disease:

Date: 10 Feb 2003

This morning I received this e-mail and then searched your archives and found nothing that pertained to it. Does anyone know anything about this problem?

[Then he quoted the text of the email:]

"Have you heard of an epidemic in Guangzhou? An acquaintance of mine from a teacher's chat room lives there and reports that the hospitals there have been closed and people are dying."

— Stephen O. Cunnion, MD, Ph.D., MPH
International Consultants in Health, Inc.
Member ASTM&H, ISTM

The same day, the World Health Organization (WHO) office in Beijing received an email message from the son of a former WHO staff member, now living in Guangdong, describing an infectious disease in the province that was said to have caused more than 100 deaths. The WHO was also finding out about the epidemic through other channels, as we'll see in the next chapter.

The WHO sent a query to Beijing, asking about this reported outbreak, and the following day, February 11, the Chinese wall of secrecy showed a small crack: the Guangzhou Bureau of Health reported to the press more than 100 cases of an outbreak of atypical pneumonia that had been spreading in the city for more than a month.

The same day, the Chinese Ministry of Health in Beijing officially reported to the WHO that some kind of respiratory illness, apparently an unidentified form of pneumonia, had struck 305 people in Guangdong province. Five had died, and 59 had recovered and subsequently been discharged. About a third of those affected were medical personnel, but none of them had died, the Ministry said—although this would turn out to be inaccurate. The majority of the cases had been discovered in Guangzhou, but others had been affected in the cities of Jiangmen, Foshan, Zhongshan and Shenzhen-all of which lie in the Pearl River Delta region around Hong Kong.

The next day the Ministry reported that the outbreak dated back to November 16, 2002, and that the disease organism had not yet been isolated, but that the outbreak was coming under control. What followed was a spate of attempts to make the situation seem more or less normal.

"This is in no way a terrifying disease and there is no need to panic," Huang Qingdao, head of the Guangdong Department of Health, told the press. "The virus only poses a danger of infection if it can accumulate in the air to a certain density, so maintaining good air circulation is very important."

"After taking effective measures, the disease has been initially brought under control," a spokesman for the Guangdong provincial government said. "The three cities of Foshan, Heyuan and Zhongshan have no more new cases reported."

At another news conference, Guangzhou Vice-Mayor Chen Chuanyu asserted that the city had world-class medical facilities, and was able to cope with any epidemic. None of the municipal party and government officials had, so far, taken anti-virus medicines and vaccines, he said, apparently as a way to bolster public morale.

A doctor who gave his surname as Lei, from an infectious disease hospital in Guangzhou, said that following investigations, hospitals had come up with the right medicines to curb the disease.

The US initially echoed this sentiment. Wendy Lyle, a spokeswoman for the U.S. Consulate in Guangzhou, said it was not offering any special advice regarding the outbreak, although it had received numerous inquiries from American citizens. "The situation is quite under control," said Lyle.

* * *

It's hard to know exactly what happened in China in the closing months of 2002. Records have been lost or were never kept; specimens were never taken or have been lost. Nobody knew, after all, that certain events were connected; nor did they know that was beginning, or how scrupulously it should be documented.

On November 16, two or three residents of Foshan, an industrial city in the Pearl River Delta with a population of some 3.5 million, came down with an unusual form of pneumonia. The first symptoms were fever and a dry cough, and in some cases also aching muscles, a sore throat, and diarrhea—just like flu, in fact. Disturbingly, however, some patients rapidly developed such difficulty breathing that they had to use ventilators to keep them alive.

Common pneumonia is an infection caused by bacteria, viruses, or fungi. Typically, you cough, your lungs fill with watery mucus, you develop a high temperature, you feel weak, and you find it hard to breathe. Inside, the causative agents spread throughout one or both of your lungs. As long as your resistance is reasonably strong, your health in general is fair, and you are treated promptly with appropriate medication (such as targeted antibiotics), you should recover in a week or two. Those who die of pneumonia are usually elderly—or in the age of AIDS, have some fragility in their immune system. Pneumonia has traditionally been called "the old man's friend," as it hastens a relatively painless exit. The SARS pneumonia was unusual—atypical, in medical language—for several reasons. The infection didn't produce the usual amounts of watery mucus; instead, the lungs tended to swell and compress against the chest, making it difficult to breathe. It was difficult for medical staff to get a sputum sample, and when they did, it didn't seem to contain any of the usual suspects. Furthermore, some patients moved with alarming speed to the stage where they were having trouble breathing and needed to be put on a ventilator. Antibiotics didn't seem to help. Many of these signs suggested that the pneumonia was being caused by a virus rather than a bacterium, but the usual antiviral medications didn't help much either. The Foshan residents died, and because pneumonia is common, their deaths passed largely unremarked.

"We did not take it seriously at the beginning," an official from the Guangdong Provincial Centre for Disease Control and Prevention told a reporter for the Toronto Globe and Mail.

More than a third of the first wave of casualties were food handlers-that is, people who raised, handled, killed or sold animals destined to be food, or chefs who subsequently killed, prepared or served food. It remains unclear if that clustering was noticed at the time, but it would turn out to be the subject of intense interest. Within a few days, more cities in Guangdong province reported this unusual pneumonia, and by December, a mild panic ensued when seven hospital staff in the city of Heyuan were found to have been infected.

For whatever reasons, this information was not passed on in response to the WHO inquiries, nor even, as far as we can tell, disseminated to other provinces. On January 3, in fact, the local health bureau announced through a Heyuan newspaper: "No epidemic disease is being spread in Heyuan... symptoms like cough and fever appear due to relatively colder weather."

The fact that any statement at all was made may be a sign that anxiety was spreading, as was the disease. According to newspaper reports published several weeks later, a pig farmer, a seafood merchant, and a 10-year-old boy all came down with atypical pneumonia. After the boy died, hospital workers posthumously nicknamed him "Du Huang" or "the Emperor of Poison." He had infected five of them, including an ambulance driver and doctor who later died. In Guangzhou, staff at the Second Affiliated Sun Yat-sen Hospital later dubbed the seafood merchant "a walking biological weapon," because he seemed to have infected everyone around him.

Meanwhile, Chinese authorities ordered journalists not to report on the outbreak. A reporter at a newspaper in Shenzhen, just across the border from Hong Kong, said the ban came even as his manager passed out Chinese herbal medicine to fight the disease.

The medical authorities in Guangdong province were neither idle nor lacking in competence. On January 23rd, an expert report on the outbreak was drawn up, and under these new and confusing circumstances it was remarkably accurate. The disease, it said, was an atypical pneumonia of unknown causes, probably viral in origin. It gave a good description of the epidemiology and clinical features, stressed the importance of infection control, and advised both alertness and caution. The report had only one major shortcoming: it was circulated only to medical institutions within the province, but not to the WHO or to its neighbor, Hong Kong.

"Neither the Hong Kong government or the WHO received the report or its detail until a later stage," said Margaret Chan Fung Fu-chun, the Hong Kong director of health during the outbreak (and at this writing, the WHO director of protection of the human environment). She said that she and her department's consultant, Tse Lai-yin, called Guangdong health authorities several times to verify reports of illness in Guangdong but were unable to reach officials. A Guangdong official later told her "there was a legal requirement for infectious diseases at that time that infectious diseases were classified as state secrets. That is why they cannot share the information."

Besides, it now seems as if the initial set of cases was confined to several small clusters, after which the outbreak apparently quieted down. Chinese officials seem to have hoped or assumed that the worst was over. Instead, the disease rebounded and began to grow dramatically during the last week of January 2003, when infected hospitalized patients spread the virus to health care workers, other patients, and visitors. One person with the virus, treated at several facilities, is thought to have infected the staggering number of 91 persons, including 79% of the staff at one hospital. The outbreak peaked during the first ten days of February, when close to 40 new cases were being reported each day. Altogether, some 1,512 cases are thought to have occurred during the Guangdong outbreak, most of them health care workers in urban hospitals.

Word of this disturbing development apparently spread within China, and some of China's other provinces immediately began to gear up for an outbreak. (The 1-billion plus population of China is no stranger to infectious disease. Quite apart from HIV/AIDS, at any given time some province in China is usually battling an outbreak of one disease or another.) Not all provinces were so alert, though; one of the areas that did little preparation was Beijing.

In late January, a provincial newspaper ran a brief statement from the authorities: "This virus has been present in Guangzhou for more than a month, and the illness of those afflicted has been effectively treated and controlled."

"There is no need for people to panic."

* * *

In both Guangdong and Hong Kong, however, people thought otherwise. Rumors spread at the speed of text messages on cell phones. One rumor said bioterrorists had struck Guangzhou's World Trade Centre building. Managers there reacted by disinfecting the whole skyscraper. Disinfectant was also reportedly sprayed in the Guangzhou city subway as well as on 6,000 public buses and 16,000 taxis.

An Australian businessman in Hong Kong called home saying that bubonic plague was on the loose. A local newspaper suspected anthrax. A Department of Health spokeswoman moved to calm fears by announcing that the government had enough smallpox vaccine to deal with a potential act of bioterrorism, though the Hong Kong Medical Association chairman doubted this, and in turn said that in the event of a biological attack the government would draw up a list of priorities with vaccines going first to high-ranking officials—a reassurance hardly likely to calm the general public.

As the news and rumors spread, so did street prevention: travelers waiting for trains at Guangzhou's railroad station, and fans watching a China-Brazil soccer match were reported to be wearing surgical masks or covering their faces with tissues. Pharmacies couldn't keep up with demand for Banlangen granule, a popular Chinese herbal medicine made from root of indigowood widely used by mainlanders as a cure for colds and fever.

"All inventories were sold out in the past few days," said a spokesman for the makers of the medication, Guangzhou Baiyunshan Pharmaceutical Corp. "In January, we sold 40,000 boxes of Banlangen granule, each with 1,000 small packs. But sales reached 7,000 boxes on the first day the news of the virus spread."

"We are producing up to 3,000 boxes a day and all have been sold. In the past two days, we worked 24 hours each day to make the drug to meet demand." The company said it was raising the wholesale price of Banlangen by 10% "due to increased demand and operating costs."

It wasn't only practitioners of traditional Chinese medicine who propagated the rumors and remedies; and the means by which rumor spread weren't just by old-fashioned gossip. On February 9, 2003, officials from the multi-national pharmaceutical company Roche held a news conference to say that since the mystery flu resembled the H5N1 avian flu that had broken out in 1997, Roche's Tamiflu anti-viral medication would be an effective treatment. As soon as the conference ended, newspapers reported, "mobile phone text messages and Internet reports repeating these claims spread across the province." Sales went so well that Roche shipped more in from its Shanghai factory.

Guangdong law-enforcement authorities warned Roche that it would be "seriously punished if it was found to have spread rumors that Guangdong was in the grip of pneumonia and bird-flu outbreak." Roche denied that it had spread rumors, saying Tamiflu sales had been strong even before the press conference.

"The sickness is not really that huge an event. It's the panic that's turning into the real epidemic," said Xu Yueheng, deputy director of the Guangdong provincial disease control center. "In this age of the Internet and instant-text messaging on everyone's mobile phone, it's gotten a whole lot worse."

Rumors spread and rebounded, producing their own sub-rumors. In Hong Kong, the word on the street was that two people had been arrested in Guangdong for using mobile phones to send messages containing rumors about an "epidemic," though police would not confirm any such arrests.

When the government did issue official advice, it was a combination of the helpful and the unhelpful. The Guangdong Department of Health urged the city's residents to maintain good air circulation in their homes, stay away from crowded areas such as shopping centers and train stations, maintain good personal hygiene, and fumigate their rooms with vinegar (regarded in traditional Chinese medicine as a germicide, and given significantly less credence in traditional Western medicine).

Throughout Guangdong, Hong Kong, and Macau, people stampeded to buy vinegar. Lines formed at stores selling bulk vinegar, with clerks using funnels to fill empty plastic soda bottles. One Chinese daily reported that the prices of surgical masks and vinegar had risen twenty-fold. A Hong Kong paper found some stores in the New Territories charging as much as HK$100 for a bottle of vinegar compared with the normal price of HK$8 before the outbreak. Share prices for drug companies and vinegar producers rose by up to 10 percent in one day.

"You go into some offices in Guangzhou, the whole damn building smells like vinegar, from the entrance to the elevator and up to the office," said Ben Mok, a Canadian who was the general manager for Coca-Cola, Inc. in northeastern China.

In Guangzhou, meanwhile, the remedy of choice was a bitter, black tea-like infusion called liang cha. Newspapers and television stations reported that Dr. Zhong Jiaxi, a researcher at Guangzhou University of Traditional Chinese Medicine, had prescribed it to a patient suffering from atypical pneumonia in Foshan in November when Western medicine didn't seem to be helping.

"At that time we didn't know much about the illness. I was asked to treat him with Chinese medicine and his fever subsided after the first dose and he fully recovered after three doses. My treatment consists of getting rid of the heat, poison and water in the body, so I prescribe herbs like honeysuckle and chrysanthemum," he said. "I want to stress that this medicine has preventive qualities but it is not 100 percent effective. It is possible that you will still fall ill after taking the medicine because there are so many factors causing the disease."

Despite this disclaimer, people began lining up for liang cha. A drugstore clerk said he had sold dozens of packages in two days. A street vendor running a liang cha stand said she had sold several kettles of the drink on Monday and Tuesday at two yuan (about 25 cents) a cup. The Guangdong International Hotel served liang cha in its restaurants. Managers at the World Trade Centre office complex offered liang cha to their tenants.

"It's one of the preventive measures we are taking to assure tenants," an employee of the building management said. "We have also fumigated the building with steaming vinegar."

By now, though, vinegar was turning out to be not only useless but potentially lethal. An 80-year-old Guangzhou man was rushed to the hospital with a "damaged digestive system" after drinking vinegar ar every meal, and in two separate incidents in Guangdong, a boy (variously reported as being six or seven years old) and a young woman of eighteen died of carbon monoxide poisoning after vinegar had been boiled in their apartments.

* * *

The Hong Kong Health Department suspected that what was happening was what they had feared since 1997: the return of avian influenza, this time as a full-blown epidemic. It took the this fog of threats and rumors seriously enough to convene, on February 11, a Working Party on what it decided to call Severe Community-Acquired Pneumonia—SCAP for short. "Community-acquired" refers to any pneumonia that developed prior to admission, rather than while the patient was already in the hospital; the SCAP group consisting of experts in microbiology, intensive care, and internal medicine which met seven times in as many days and made two recommendations that would turn out to be both wise and timely.

The first was that, effective immediately, all hospitals were required to report any suspicious and severe pneumonias to the Department of Health at once.

The second, issued on February 21st, was that when dealing with suspected cases of the atypical pneumonia, health care staff were instructed to wear N95 masks—that is, masks designed to filter out 95% of particles larger than 0.3 microns in diameter. (Individual viruses are smaller than 0.3 microns, but they tend to cluster.) They were also instructed to wear gowns and to use certain other anti-infection measures. As things would turn out, SCAP issued this order not a moment too soon.

Chapter 3.

GOARN—Global Outbreak and Response Network

In addition to Fred Leung, the Hong Kong Health Department, and the Guangdong medical establishment, a number of interested parties outside China were watching for signs of flu, avian or otherwise. What was about to happen was later described by Dr. David Heymann, then Executive Director for Communicable Diseases for the WHO, as "a roll out" for a global disease surveillance and response system that had been in the making for a decade or more.

In 1991, after more than a century's absence, epidemic cholera struck Latin America, infecting 400,000 people and killing 4,000 within a year. In 1994, plague broke out in Surat, India; the following year, Ebola hemorrhagic fever struck in the Congo, an outbreak that took everyone by surprise. Heymann saw this epidemic firsthand he was there as an epidemiologist—and when he returned to WHO headquarters in Geneva he carried with him the conviction that the world needed a reliable early-warning system for infectious diseases.

In fact, four interlocking early-warning systems developed, of which the first was GOARN: the Global Outbreak Alert and Response Network. GOARN started as a coalition founded in 1997, and consisting of the 141 WHO country offices concentrated in the developing world, as well as more than 110 existing institutes, laboratories, agencies, and surveillance systems from around the world, with a wide range of expertise in infectious diseases. GOARN's job would be to share incoming information, pool resources and expertise, and try to address the fact that a major infectious disease outbreak would be a global problem needing a global effort to contain it.

The two principal figures in the GOARN office at the WHO were Drs. David Heymann and Guenael Rodier.

Heymann was a veteran of both public health and outbreaks of infectious disease. After finishing medical school, he went to the London School of Hygiene & Tropical Medicine, got recruited into the smallpox eradication program in the seventies, then worked for CDC for 25 years in international activities, the last five years seconded to WHO. Even behind a desk as one of the senior most individuals in global public health, he has the lean build and greyhound intensity of a man who has been out in the field and never really come back.

"When I started at CDC in 1976 my first assignment was what was thought to be a swine flu outbreak in Philadelphia which turned out to be Legionnaire's Disease. My second was to Ebola in Zaire, which was a new virus, and after that I went to Africa and stayed for thirteen years there as an epidemiologist." With this background he found himself in the mid-1990s working for the WHO on HIV/AIDS and eventually, heading all communicable disease activities. (After the SARS outbreak, his career trajectory would take him back to disease eradication, as a senior advisor to the WHO director-general on polio eradication.)

Rodier, though also a field veteran, is Heymann's counterpart and opposite: younger and more voluble, with a surfeit of energy and high spirits, he has the look of a man who went off to a Nouvelle Vague film series ten years ago and hasn't stopped talking since. (Around WHO, Rodier's first name is pronounced "G'nell," as if the speaker were an Australian greeting an orange seller.) He was born in Africa, went back to Africa, and worked five years as a GP in Djibouti, almost entirely in infectious diseases and pediatrics. Then, like Heymann, he studied tropical medicine in London, moved to the US Navy out of Cairo studying infectious disease threat assessment, and after four years joined the WHO. In 1994, during India's plague outbreak, Rodier was in Copenhagen when he got a call inviting him to take the next plane to Geneva so he could accompany the Director General to India and work on infectious disease surveillance. Following his experience with plague in India, plus stints working on Ebola in Zaire, Heymann approached him to work on the epidemic response team. The cast was being assembled.

The third figure who needs introducing at this point is Dr. Michael Ryan, a red-headed Irishman built like a stack of bricks, but with a quick mind and the unusual ability to combine scientific articulation and explosive humor in the same sentence.

"In 1994-95 we had the outbreak of Ebola in Kikwit, and David went there because he had previous Ebola experience—he was in the global program on AIDS at the time. And he was joined in the field by Guenael, who at the time was working in [Information Technology] here [in Geneva], but Guenael had a background in Africa, spoke French, knew the score, so he got sent out there with a few of the boys.

"When they came back there was this new unit created called Emerging Diseases, and various people were popped into the unit, but what you had was a smorgasbord of individual disease experts in the classic WHO sense of the word. WHO had its experts on this and its experts on that, and they had expert meetings every so often and produced guidelines and did lab science, and that's a very important role for WHO. But what we didn't have was the operational capacity to assist countries in the middle of an epidemic. And David wanted that.

"I wasn't here at the time—I came over in '96. I went in to meet David and Guenael and walked out thinking, 'Oh, God.' I could feel destiny. I joined three weeks later, and I spent 33 weeks in the field each year for the next four years. Along with some other fellows, I just got thrown at the outbreaks. David wanted to regain credibility for the WHO, and the only way we were going to do that was out there. Ebola, meningitis, cholera, shigella, relapsing fever, Rift Valley fever—Christ almighty! A wing and a prayer, no security. . .

"We gradually began to reengage with CDC, Institut Pasteur, MSF [Medecins Sans Frontieres, or Doctors Without Borders] and all these other players; we were beginning to work together in the field and find our way in the field, dealing with logistics, dealing with security. Some successes, some failures, and lots of tension in the field!"

These were the birthing pains of David Heymann's small, light, and cheap "rapid response force" to deal with emerging infectious diseases. This force, it must be stressed, no more consisted of WHO staffers than a U.N. peacekeeping force consists of Geneva bureaucrats. What the WHO was starting to learn to do was act by what can be considered the Heymann Doctrine: identify resources all over the globe and bring them together to where they were needed.

"We were starting to see that everyone had a role to play," Ryan went on. "MSF can do brilliant logistics and they can put up a bloody hospital in two days. CDC—wonderful investigators. Institut Pasteur has the language skills, and they're based in Africa. There was this realization that if we could work together we'd have this virtual CDC for the world. That's really where the whole idea for the network came from—that experience in the field, just grinding it out. We knew that we needed a better logistics platform, a better security platform, a better environment in which teams could work, and the WHO could provide that. We have access to the countries, or most of them—we've got that mandate to be there.

"That came to fruition in April 2000, with the first meeting of the network. We all sat around, we had a great meeting, we talked about this and that. May, June, the summer came, we wrote some documents, we thought this was a great idea, and then, bang! October. Ebola in Uganda. And we had to put this [idea] into practice.

"I went into the field on October 2nd and came back on January 15th, two weeks before my kid was born, so I was gone for the last four months of my wife's pregnancy," he sighed. "And we were out there burying the bodies and doing everything... but the thing that happened was that there was a fundamental shift. We had tensions in the field, but for once we provided the platform. We worked with the Red Cross, MSF, and twenty-two different organizations in the field in a very complex environment, security-wise [in other words, in the middle of a civil war]. For me, the meeting in April was neither here nor there. Ebola in Uganda created the network."

That last point bears repeating: with the right vision and will, the necessity of responding to outbreaks give birth to the invention—the means to control outbreaks. Much as the body's immune response is shaped and refined by exposure to infection, what Heymann was trying to create was, in effect, a global immune system.

* * *

The network needed pertinent, accurate, timely information—and while WHO still relied on getting information from the governments of member nations, this information tended to be incomplete and/or very slow in coming.

With this in mind, the epidemic response team got very interested in the Global Public Health Intelligence Network (GPHIN, pronounced "giffen"), developed by Health Canada. GPHIN was a web-crawling service that tracked more than 950 news feeds, wire services, and open medical sites such as ProMED, discussion groups, and bulletin boards, searching for disease news and information by keywords. At the time of the SARS outbreak it searched in English and French; since then, Russian, Chinese, Spanish, and Arabic have been added, at least in part because of the overlap between epidemic disease and bioterrorism.

GPHIN's premise was that diseases could be circulating long before any official report was made to the WHO—or to anyone, in fact. According to the British medical journal The Lancet, about 65% of the world's first news of infectious disease events now comes from informal sources, including press reports and the Internet. And when ProMED began trading questions and rumors about the "strange contagious disease" with respiratory symptoms that was killing health workers in Guangdong hospitals and causing "widespread panic," word was passed on at once to the WHO.

Simultaneously, the U.S. Department of Defense's Global Emerging Infections Surveillance and Response System (DoD-GEIS), was also carrying out surveillance. GEIS, another web-crawling system founded by US President Clinton in 1996, has a specific brief to watch for diseases that might affect military personnel, and to coordinate the efforts of various military laboratories and facilities so as to reduce that risk. GEIS, too, picked up reports about a severe outbreak in Beijing and Guangzhou, but the suspected cause was identified as influenza B.

Tracking and assessing all this information was the WHO Influenza Laboratory Network of 100 labs in 84 countries, set up in 1948 to track flu viruses and coordinate the international response, including advice on preparing vaccines. This is a crucial task since flu vaccines need to be prepared several months ahead of the coming flu season. As each outbreak may involve different flu strains, it is essential for, say, the CDC in Atlanta to know which strains of flu are raging in Hong Kong one winter so they can add their antibody to the US vaccine for the following winter.

"There are probably about fifty infectious disease outbreaks reported to us each year," Heymann said—roughly one a week. Of all the diseases being watched for in China by these networks, the prime suspect, and also the most feared, was flu.

On 23 November 2002, during a routine flu workshop in China attended by a WHO scientist, a participant from Guangdong Province reported on a "serious outbreak with high mortality and involvement of health care staff." On 27 November, GPHIN picked up rustlings and murmurings of a "flu outbreak" in mainland China.

Despite its high-tech surveillance systems and its new epidemic response team, the WHO was in an awkward position. As a United Nations agency, it cannot intervene in the affairs of any country unless invited; conversely, the only diseases that a country was required to report to the WHO at the time, as set out in the International Health Regulations, were plague, cholera, and yellow fever.

A query was passed via WHO office in Beijing to the Chinese health authorities. Nothing was heard back until December, when a confirmation of sorts was made: yes, there had been an outbreak of Influenza B, but it was nothing out of the ordinary, and now was under control. That was it.

Chapter 4.

Too Many Viruses

On February 19, nine days after word began to leak out of Guangdong, China, about the strange pneumonia, and the equally strange epidemic of vinegar-boiling, the World Health Organization issued a global health alert that would turn out to be yet another red herring. It was for bird flu.

A Hong Kong family had gone on vacation to the coastal province of Fujian, the next coastal province north of Guangdong, at the end of January, and one by one started falling seriously ill. The daughter, aged eight, died in Fujian of pneumonia. The rest of the family was hurried back to Hong Kong, but the father died, despite extensive treatment. The mother developed a flu-like viral condition but recovered. The son, aged nine, was found to be infected with H5N1 virus—the first case of avian influenza contracted by a human since the deadly outbreak in 1997. It wasn't clear, either, how the family had caught the virus. Although living and hygiene conditions in the area were generally poor, and drinking water was drawn from a well, apparently none of the family members in Fujian were suffering from pneumonia nor the bird flu.

Other relatives said the family had spent the night of January 31 at a squatter hut near the ancestral home. The little girl began coughing, and the following day, when the whole family was at the ancestral home, she started to vomit and suffered chest pains. She was admitted to a local hospital on February 3, and died of pneumonia the following day.

Relatives said they later collected her body from the hospital for burial on a hillside near the ancestral home. They said the father looked tired after his daughter was taken ill but did not display any flu symptoms.

Health officials in Fujian also denied that the family could have contracted pneumonia or the bird flu in their area. "We believe the girl did not contract the virus in our province," the spokesman for the Fujian Provincial Public Health Department said yesterday. "Our investigations show that none of the 65 people who came into contact with the girl has developed any symptoms of flu or pneumonia."

To add to the sense of combined alarm and denial, Guangzhou residents watching news about the avian flu on television stations out of Hong Kong found that the transmission was abruptly cut off.

"I heard the news on Hong Kong television news last night but the transmission was interrupted midway," a businesswoman told a local paper. "I tend to think it's H5N1 because a friend who is a nurse told us so. You can't believe the government because they cover up a lot of things."

Chen Jiasheng, a senior protocol officer at the Guangdong foreign affairs office, denied that the government had intercepted the television signals.

"This is not government behavior. The government did not order a news blackout. Some overzealous television official probably took it upon himself to block the broadcast because he thought it was sensitive."

Still, the deaths had undoubtedly been caused by H5N1 virus, and on February 19 the matter was reported to the WHO Influenza Laboratory Network by the Hong Kong Department of Health. The WHO alert summarized the events, concluding:

"It is not yet known whether the other family members who fell ill were also infected with A (H5N1). A medical and epidemiological investigation is ongoing in Hong Kong SAR to determine the cause of those illnesses and deaths, and results should be available in the next few days. Investigations are also ongoing to determine the source of the infection.

"The World Health Organization is collaborating closely with health authorities in Beijing and Hong Kong SAR. The WHO Global Influenza Surveillance Network has been alerted and WHO has offered to provide support if required."

The timing of the avian influenza infections was exquisitely strange. There hadn't been a case of human avian influenza in five years, and now it appeared at a time when it couldn't possibly have been more dramatic, or more misleading.

"Everyone, from WHO down, was expecting a [flu] pandemic," explained Dr. Lo Su Vui, the Head of the Hong Kong Health Department's research office. "Pandemics occur every thirty to forty years. The question is not whether, but when." The mysterious disease in Guangdong, plus these clearly identified cases from Fujian, fitted together perfectly: the expected influenza pandemic was breaking, and it was H5N1 avian influenza virus.

To confuse matters further, other pneumonias were rife. On January 24th it was announced that a ten-year-old-boy and his 77-year-old grandfather had died of flu in the Prince of Wales Hospital. The boy developed septicemia; the grandfather, who already suffered from chronic lung disease and had survived a stroke, died of pneumonia. It turned out the fatal virus had not been imported from mainland China; it had been picked up in Japan. The boy's parents, a domestic helper, and a family friend had been on vacation in Hokkaido, where they contracted the virus and took it back home to China. It swept through the family, affecting everyone. The grandparents and grandchildren were hit hardest, and were rushed to hospital. The grandmother and the boy's two younger siblings recovered; the grandfather and the boy died.

This event, tragic though it was, would turn out to be yet another red herring. The fatal agent was neither bird flu nor SARS—it was a rogue flu variant that to all intents and purposes came out of nowhere and after this single distressing appearance, vanished.

At the same time, the Hong Kong Department of Health found a sharp rise in respiratory infections caused by adenovirus and influenza B virus—leading to, among other outcomes, pneumonia. Infections caused by adenovirus jumped from 25 cases in August 2002 to 84 cases in December, while influenza B infections rose from just three cases to 67 over the same period.

But influenza was just one of the possibilities that was suggested as a cause of the mysterious outbreak in Guangdong. One Hong Kong rumor said it was naturally-occurring anthrax, originating on the mainland. Beijing announced that chlamydia was the cause (the chlamydia variant causing pneumonia is a relative of the sexually transmitted version). Other suggestions, more and less professional in origin, ranged from the somewhat unlikely to the downright arcane. They included leptospirosis (a bacterial animal disease—i.e., a zoonosis—usually transmitted to humans by exposure to water contaminated by animal urine), Legionnaire's disease (a cause of pneumia initially isolated in the US during a Legionnaire's convention), pulmonary plague, and hemorrhagic fever.

On top of all this, pneumonia is a common enough disease to cause extra confusion. In any given month in Hong Kong, well over a thousand people come down with some form of pneumonia. In the period of February 1-26, 2003 alone, 39 people turned up at a hospital with severe community-acquired pneumonia—and to make matters still more confusing, over a third had recently traveled to China, and nearly two-thirds turned out to be suffering from a pneumonia of unknown origin that was not SARS.

In the military intelligence business, it is said, the main problem consists of separating the signal from the background noise. With so many disparate and scattered pieces of information coming in from so many sources, which is important? Which connects to other pieces? Which is potentially lethal? When SARS finally appeared it did so in disguise, concealed behind this hubbub of viral information.

* * *

Yet whether the emerging outbreak was avian flu, or some other virulent flu, or a new virus altogether, it was emerging in time-honored fashion at a time-honored destination (or transit point, as it turned out): Hong Kong.

Its location means that time and again Hong Kong has been hit by outbreaks of infectious disease; yet for that very reason, it has become a major center for studying and combating those infections.

Modern Hong Kong is a successful world city on a scale that makes Manhattan seem old, dingy, and roomy. Not only are there more than 6 million people living in 1100 square kilometers, but most of that acreage is uninhabitably steep, or consists of small uninhabited islands. The small amount of available land, then, is packed with skyscrapers routinely rising thirty floors or more. This density reduces traffic arteries to mere capillaries. Traffic barely moves; the only efficient way to get around is by the quick, clean MTR subway system, the double-decker buses and small, speedy, apparently outlaw minibuses. This is a city of collective public spaces, like so many of the vast, modern, growing cities of the East. Coming into Hong Kong at evening rush hour from Macau, ferry passengers wait in a mass ten abreast and fifty to a hundred deep to enter the immigration and arrivals hall. The prevalent school of architecture is the mall; the state flower is the escalator. Unlike Americans, isolated in their cars, the denizens of Hong Kong rub shoulders in enclosed spaces several hours a day. It's a virus's paradise.

On the other hand, Hong Kong is anything but a teeming mass of huddled humanity. As a city, it is remarkably clean, neat, orderly, and well-run. It also has a long tradition of studying, treating, and guarding against infectious disease. The University of Hong Kong Medical School was founded in 1887 by Dr. (Sir) Patrick Manson. Manson was by no coincidence a microbiologist, a parasitologist, and is regarded as the father of tropical medicine. He discovered the cause of elephantiasis (lymphatic filariasis) and was the first to argue that malaria was transmitted by mosquitoes.

In 1894, Hong Kong suffered its first outbreak of plague, and at once became a focal point for such intensive and skilled research that the plague bacillus was identified and studied for the first time.

Professor Kwok-Yung Yuen, Head of the Department of Microbiology and Chair of Infectious Disease at the University of Hong Kong, explained the connection of Honk Kong with the flu. "In 1957, we had an outbreak of Asian flu in Hong Kong. In 1968 we had an outbreak of Hong Kong flu. These caused pandemics."

In some Western minds, this association with influenza suggests that flu epidemics are somehow Hong Kong's fault, and must be caused by conditions in Hong Kong. In Hong Kong, though, the city is seen (with considerable pride) as the first line of defense—a forward observer, perhaps, in a foxhole ahead of the front lines—against infectious disease emerging in the entire East Asian region, and South China in particular.

"It's not that Hong Kong is dirtier," Yuen went on. "It's because Hong Kong has a much better infrastructure than China. We have a much better public health and research infrastructure, so many of these agents are first found in Hong Kong. They don't originate in Hong Kong. We have been protecting the world for a long time, actually."

In February 2003, nobody realized that Hong Kong was poised to play a curious double-role in world health: it was about to act as a launching point for the first major global epidemic of the twenty-first century; and once again it was about to do more than its share of work to protect the world from that epidemic.

Chapter 5.

Global Warning, Global Alarm

The world in general, of course, knew nothing about what was happening in Hong Kong. If there was any emerging infectious disease on the radar screen it was Ebola, which the WHO confirmed on February 19th had broken out in the Congo. Yet that outbreak didn't make the front pages: by now Ebola had broken out several times without sweeping the planet, and despite being a very nasty disease with a book (The Hot Zone) and a movie (Outbreak) to its name, it was rapidly becoming old news.

However, on the same date the WHO issued its avian influenza alert, and this was something new. As a result, the alert had the largely unintended effect of redefining the outbreak: it was no longer a local threat but a global one.

While the confusing events concerning both the lethal atypical pneumonia and the bird flu had been confined to the Far East, coverage in the West had been perfunctory. Anxiety seemed confined to the same area as the disease. (One curious feature of the coverage is that one country's newspaper was all too ready to say that another country was panicking, it took a substantial degree of alarm-raising before anyone would diagnose panic in their own backyard.)

Over the week after the WHO alert, though, it was as if the world was swept by a global epidemic of alarm. Instead of the new avian influenza/atypical pneumonia being compared to the 1997 Hong Kong avian flu epidemic, which had little meaning for most of the world, it was now compared to epidemics of far greater scope.

On February 24, Gwynne Dyer, an independent journalist and historian perhaps best known for a controversial CBC series on the history of war, wrote his regular column, this time on the subject "A Plague May be Stalking Us." Dyer summarized the avian influenza deaths, reminded readers of the 1997 outbreak, then moved up a notch: "[O]nce in a while, something really lethal comes along. This could be one of those times." The "Spanish flu" pandemic of 1918, he went on, "infected between 20 and 40 per cent of the world's population and killed 20 million people in four months, twice as many as died in World War I." Bird flu, he said, could similarly cause millions of deaths.

"Nor is that the worst that could happen," he said, shifting into top gear. "Two years ago, professors Christopher Duncan and Susan Scott, of Liverpool University, suggested in their book, *Biology of Plagues*, that the Black Death was an Ebola-like virus, a haemorrhagic fever transmitted directly from person to person. It is frighteningly plausible."

He summarized the mortality statistics of the two great plague pandemics, one in 541 A.D., the other—the Black Death—in the fourteenth century, which "killed between 30 and 40 per cent of the population in the first onslaught."

"If Duncan and Scott are right," he concluded, "a virus is lying dormant while it tries out mutations that might break through the genetic defenses that human beings evolved to defeat it last time. When it does this, it could kill a significant portion of the human race in a year. The Black Death is not dead, it's only sleeping. And in the meantime, 'bird flu' may be coming."

Over the next few days, the column was reprinted in papers from Nova Scotia, Prince Edward Island, Ontario, England, New Zealand, and Australia.

At the same time, Global News Wire from the South African Press Association quoted Medinfo, an online medical advice site: "Scientists anxiously awaiting the results of tests on the boy are extremely concerned that the deadly strain of bird flu to which [the] family has fallen victim could be about to start a pandemic... indeed, many health authorities around the globe believe that another worldwide flu pandemic is already brewing."

Referring again to the epidemic of 1918, Medinfo continued, "The question is therefore not whether such an epidemic would be repeated, but when... WHO's response to this is indicative of the level of concern internationally. A flu pandemic of whatever type would be devastating for the entire world—millions will die."

These effusions of hysteria are very useful; not because their arguments hold water, which they generally don't, but because they illustrate the way in which many of us have been encouraged to think about the threat of infectious disease.

Especially since the publication of Richard Preston's book *The Hot Zone* (loosely adapted as the film *Outbreak*), infectious disease has become a sexy horror topic. Whether it be SARS, avian influenza, or, in recent years, the threat of a global Ebola outbreak or mass attacks of bioterror involving smallpox, anthrax or other pathogens, outbreaks are to the turn of the millennium what sharks (courtesy of Jaws and its ilk) were to the Seventies.

(In case this seems a fanciful analogy, this is what one reviewer wrote about Outbreak: "You have to respect viruses. These things are the killer sharks of the microscopic world, insidious, darn near indestructible little buggers who destroy every cell in their path.")

Yet Dyer's column, and the editorials of a hundred others after him, demonstrated a paradox that would be repeated over and over again during the outbreak: the farther away from the virus people were, the more afraid they were. The least afraid were those at greatest risk. This was also true of journalists: the best coverage of the outbreak came from the South China Morning Post of Hong Kong and the Straits Times of Singapore, who were right in there with everyone else.

* * *

Outside the realm of Hollywood, then, what is really going on in the world of emerging infectious diseases? What are the outbreaks we should know about?

Infectious disease is well worth taking seriously, but it consists of a number of very different threats, each with its own causes, locations, even its own season.

Some infectious diseases are the result of the fact that the world's population more than doubled in the second half of the twentieth century, accelerating most rapidly in the developing countries of the tropics and sub-tropics, where infectious diseases have long had their most tenacious hold. Population growth, rural-urban migration, and the inadequacy of sanitation and other basic infrastructures contributed to the resurgence of tuberculosis, cholera, typhoid, and plague that thrive on conditions of poor hygiene and overcrowding. Cholera, for example, has caused epidemics over the past decade in parts of Latin America where it had previously been reported only sporadically. It has split into at least two recognizable types, each with its own peculiarities and predilections to place and season. In addition, cholera has been linked with changing climate patterns and subsequently altered reservoir characteristics. While diarrheal diseases such as cholera and some types of hepatitis are spread by the so-called "fecal-oral" route, others such as malaria and yellow fever need an infected intermediate (a "vector") to do the job. Here again, countries in Africa and South America have seen a dramatic re-emergence of yellow fever since the 1980s, and forms of malaria resistant to chloroquine have become more common than susceptible forms.

In wealthier parts of the world, microbes have been quick to exploit populations made vulnerable by poverty, illness, social marginalization, or collapsing health systems. In New York City in the 1980s, multidrug-resistant strains of tuberculosis gained their hold in hospitals, prisons, and homeless populations. It served as a grim reminder that tuberculosis lies dormant in much of the world's population, needing only an immune compromise—of the body or the society—to take on an active form. Tuberculosis, including multi-drug-resistant forms, grew like a weed in the fractured countries of the former Soviet Union and re-emerged, with cases more than doubling in less than seven years. When the public health structure collapsed and immunization coverage broke down, epidemics of diphtheria returned to Russia and the Ukraine.

Human invasion of the rain forest and other wilderness areas have made it much easier for diseases that were previously confined to animals, to jump the species barrier: Lassa fever in West Africa, and hantavirus in North America among others. Chagas' disease emerged as an important human disease after mismanagement of deforested land caused populations of triatomine (a large bloodsucking insect also known as the kissing bug) to move from their wild natural hosts to involve human beings and domestic animals in the transmission cycle, eventually transforming the disease into an urban infection that can be transmitted by blood transfusion.

Excessive rainfall or drought also shift the human-animal balance—for example, by increasing the number of breeding sites for mosquitoes and moving them nearer towns and villages. In 1998 Japanese encephalitis broke out in Papua, New Guinea, when drought led to increased mosquito breeding as rivers dried into stagnant pools. The virus is now widespread in Papua, New Guinea, and threatening to move farther east. Though intensive research has failed to disclose the origins of Marburg and Ebola hemorrhagic fever outbreaks, both are thought to have animal vectors somewhere in the transmission cycle. In fact, the Ebola epidemic in the Congo that broke out at the same time as SARS would result in 80 reported cases, with 64 deaths.

In the case of influenza viruses, the most alarming recent developments are the intensive farming practices that have placed people in close proximity to domestic animals in densely populated areas. The WHO singles out the combination of "heavy international traffic, crowded conditions, and live poultry markets" of Hong Kong that contributed to the 1997 avian flu outbreak.

Other new opportunities can be attributed to the world's relaxed vigilance. After the deterioration of Aedes aegypti mosquito control campaigns during the 1970s, dengue fever resurged dramatically. Before 1970, only nine countries had experienced epidemics of dengue. Since then the number has increased more than fourfold, and continues to rise. The 1998 pandemic, in which 1-2 million cases were reported from 56 countries, was unprecedented. The resurgence of African trypanosomiasis (sleeping sickness, transmitted by the tsetse fly), which began in the 1980s, likewise followed the decline of most control activities.

Epidemics of dengue and yellow fever have been fueled by the adoption of "modern" consumer habits in urban areas of the developing world, where discarded household appliances, tires, plastic food containers and jars have created artificial breeding sites for mosquitoes and other insects. Aedes aegypti is now established in most, if not all, large African cities, greatly increasing the risk of explosive urban outbreaks. In countries of the former Soviet Union, large amounts of stagnant water, created by ineffective irrigation schemes, encouraged the re-emergence of malaria (transmitted by the Anopheles species of mosquito) in the most southern states. Tajikistan reported a few incidental cases in the early 1990s, but almost 20,000 cases in 1998.

Finally, while outbreaks of infectious disease were once thought to be the problem of poor and developing countries, that's no longer true: foot-and-mouth and mad cow disease have both caused chaos in even the most developed nations. Likewise, advances in food production and storage technology, along with the globalization of markets, have set up a food chain that is unprecedented in length and complexity—a perfect vehicle for pathogens to spread to new areas and susceptible hosts. Tracing the origin of all ingredients in a meal has become virtually impossible; controlling foodborne diseases, then, gets steadily more difficult. Nobody is safe from infectious outbreaks, and no one entity or nation can boast the tools or the expertise to quash an outbreak without difficulty.

This list, it should be borne in mind, is misleading in that the real threats to life are infectious diseases against which people could get immunized, but don't: flu, which kills 36,000 Americans each year; the millions of illnesses of childhood which Western countries provide vaccines for, but many developing countries cannot; and preventable infections that kill millions of people every year, due to lack of access to treatment available to the well-off in the West: HIV/AIDS, malaria, tuberculosis. This does not even begin to talk about the non-infectious (at least in the traditional sense) diseases of gun violence, smoking, cardiovascular disease, and many cancers.

Set out in this fashion, large-scale outbreaks of infectious disease seem curiously prosaic, the result of failures of funding or political will rather than the work of some shady bioterrorist or malign mutant virus.

This is the crux of the nightmare vision of global pandemic: it is terrifying because in nightmares we are helpless and alone.

In fact, the nightmare of pandemic disease may be frightening precisely because we don't know and can't imagine who or what stands between us and annihilation. That's hardly surprising: most Americans have a fairly good idea what doctors and nurses do, but not much about what public health really is. If anyone ever tried to sit us down and explain the infrastructures of public health and its interaction with medicine, we'd glaze over in moments.

Yet SARS proved that people were neither helpless nor alone. Ordinary people, guided and helped by local, national, and global public health and medical workers, faced a new, unknown, incurable, lethal disease, capable of infecting everyone in a room in minutes, and first contained it—at a cost, to be sure, and not without making mistakes—and then snuffed it out. For the time being, at least.

Chapter 6.

At the Metropole

While the world was worrying about bird flu and other, shadowier but more terrifying epidemics, a senior physician named Dr. Liu Jianlun and his wife took a bus from Guangzhou to Hong Kong on February 21 and checked into the three-star Hotel Metropole in Mongkok, a district of Hong Kong between the northern residential suburbs and the business and hotel district on Hong Kong Island to the south.

Dr. Liu, 64, had been working at the Second Affiliated Hospital of Sun Yat-Sen University in Guangzhou, where perhaps 45 people had been admitted with the new atypical pneumonia. He had been working long and hard on these puzzling cases, but his nephew was about to get married in Hong Kong, and although he wasn't feeling well, he didn't want to miss the wedding.

By the time Dr. Liu arrived at the Metropole, he was suffering from a high fever and a dry cough. The desk clerk assigned Dr. Liu and his wife a room on the ninth floor—by a bizarre coincidence, room 911.

In retrospect it seems almost incredible that a physician who had been treating patients with an unknown and often fatal infectious disease, and who himself was feeling unwell, would travel to one of the most densely crowded cities in the world. The fact that he did so reveals or suggests several important things about the outbreak, about SARS, and about treating infectious disease in general.

First, Professor Liu was by no means the only physician to underestimate SARS. SARS could cause as little as a passing fever and a slight cough in its first week and still be fatal. Its symptoms would often turn out to be less noticeable and disabling than symptoms of other, less serious diseases the patient was suffering at the same time. SARS was a disease that repeatedly and effectively hid behind a mask.

Second, for a resident of mainland China, especially from the province of Guangdong, travel to Hong Kong was not considered a big deal. Before the end of the twentieth century, it might have taken a Chinese citizen several years to obtain an exit visa to travel outside mainland China. Now, with Hong Kong reverting to Chinese rule and the steady opening of China to the outside world, vacationing Chinese flood into the casinos of Macau and the hotels of Hong Kong. A decade ago, China kept not only its disease statistics to itself but, to some extent, its diseases as well. Opening China let AIDS in more easily, and let SARS out more easily. Free trade breeds free trade in infection as well: over the next few weeks at least six and perhaps as many as a dozen people apart from Professor Liu would bring the virus across the porous border from the mainland into Hong Kong.

Remarkably, Liu wasn't even Hong Kong's first SARS case, though this fact was not recognized until considerably later. On January 31st, a 49-year-old woman we'll call Ms. Chang left Hong Kong to visit her mother in Henan, one of the SARS-affected cities in Guangdong. She developed a cough, then chills and a fever, and on February 17th decided to go back home and check into Union Hospital, a private hospital in Sha Tin, a district in the New Territories, near the Prince of Wales Hospital. The Hong Kong working party on community-acquired pneumonia had not yet issued its guidelines on infection control, and Ms. Chang was placed in a twin room in the medical ward, and the nursing staff wore only paper surgical masks. Two days later, having difficulty breathing, she was transferred to an isolation room, and then to the Prince of Wales Hospital, where she steadily improved. Both hospitals were amazingly lucky—only one Union Hospital nurse was infected, and she recovered. This would continue to be a characteristic of the virus: its capriciousness. On another occasion, one person sitting quietly in the corner of a room for less than three-quarters of an hour would infect more than a dozen people, some of whom merely passed through. This capriciousness, this huge discrepancy between the outcome of one potentially infectious situation and another, has never been fully explained.

The difference between Professor Liu and these other arrivals was that he stayed at a hotel. They were going home or visiting relatives. Any infections they passed on remained very local: the particular characteristic of the virus was that the person infected (usually) didn't begin to shed virus—that is, they didn't tend to breathe, cough, sneeze, or defecate it out—until they were already feeling sick enough to visit a hospital. It thus tended to engender what the medical trade calls "nosocomial" (hospital-acquired) outbreaks. A virus like

HIV/AIDS, by contrast, can infect others for years before the carrier is sick enough to need hospitalization. The dozen or so SARS-infected people apart from Liu crossed the border into residential Kowloon or the New Territories, where they would add to the growth of the Hong Kong outbreak, but nothing more.

Not only did Professor Liu stay at a hotel, but he stayed at a particular kind of hotel, that to its own misfortune and everyone else's was the perfect launch pad for the virus, to accelerate it beyond its local budding to blossom in the world at large.

The Metropole is a nice enough hotel for international guests to feel at home here, with its shuttle service and its business suite, and at any given time it hosts guests from probably a dozen different nations. It isn't the most expensive or prestigious hotel in Hong Hong (nor is it in a prime location, Kowloon being a little like Brooklyn to Hong Kong Island's Manhattan), but that is, in fact, the point. If it had been at the very top of the international class, a doctor from mainland China could never have afforded to stay there. Equally, if it had been smaller or shabbier, international visitors to Hong Kong would turn up their noses at it, and the virus would never have got out of Hong Kong. So the Metropole fit the profile: Hong Kong offered the virus a gateway to the world; the blameless and unfortunate Metropole launched it out of that gate.

Three more points might be made in passing: (1) At the time, Continental Airlines was offering a package deal to Hong Kong that included a three-night stay at the Metropole. (2) The Metropole is a favorite destination for tour parties from mainland China because the owner of the Metropole is from China. (3) In the aftermath of the SARS outbreak, health officials in Hong Kong thought long and hard about ways to get early information that would let them know that an outbreak was beginning. They even considered requiring practitioners of esoteric and traditional Chinese medicine to report possible cases to the Health Department. But as far as one can tell, nobody considered requiring health reports from hotels. When health authorities in Hong Kong started the process of contact tracing (that is, trying to find out everyone who came in contact with an infectious person, to find out who infected them, and who they in turn may have infected) the Metropole, like most hotels, had almost no information on its guests or their subsequent movements. And they had no record at all of anyone who visited the hotel's guests in their rooms—a factor that would turn out to be crucial. Hotels are perfect transit stations for infectious disease.

Dr Liu's stay in room 911 of the Metropole lasted just one night, but in that time he unwittingly passed the virus on to at least 16 other hotel guests and visitors. All of these sixteen stayed on or had a connection to the ninth floor. Over the next few days the 16 carried the virus with them as they went into local hospitals or flew to Singapore, Canada, and Viet Nam. In the words of the WHO, "An international outbreak that eventually spread to 30 countries had thus been seeded."

* * *

While this is true, it's still unclear how Dr. Liu unintentionally infected so many people—and why he infected people at the Metropole but seemingly not at the wedding banquet he went to with his wife that evening.

One early theory considered elevators: he might have coughed or sneezed while in an elevator or waiting for one, infecting those around him. This seems unlikely: based on personal experience, it's challenging to fit more than six or seven people into one of the four elevators at the Metropole, and they're sufficiently efficient that it's hard to imagine sixteen people plus Dr. Liu all waiting on the ninth floor at the same time. The virus can survive for some time outside the body, though, and this led to the possibility that Dr. Liu touched elevator button number 9, depositing some virus which was then picked up by others who touched the same button and then touched their mouth, or nose, or eyes. This is in turn led to a fear throughout the province of infected surfaces in general and elevator buttons in particular. It seems highly unlikely, though, that sixteen people could each pick up enough virus from the button without smearing it clean—or if there was such a load of virus that this mechanism was possible, why did others over the next few days remain immune?

Other theories considered air conditioning—but why would that only circulate virus on the ninth floor? A final culprit was the carpeting: what if he coughed or sneezed virus into the carpeting—perhaps in the elevator area—and the hotel vacuum cleaner sucked it up and atomized it in an aerosol that would hang in the air for much longer than the larger droplet form? Weeks later, a WHO investigative team would find viral material in the carpet, and develop the hypothesis that Professor Liu vomited in the corridor and broadcast the virus in this way—but if that were true, how come the hotel staff who cleaned it up were not infected? The whole scenario remains a mystery—and as such it developed its own ominous power in people's imagination.

* * *

On February 22, Dr. Liu walked less than a quarter of a mile down Waterloo Road from the Metropole to the Accident and Emergency Department of Kwong Wah Hospital, a modest-sized but modern urban hospital, and sought treatment for fever, shortness of breath, and palpitations.

Dr. Chow Kin-wa, the medical resident on call, said Liu told him he had been suffering from fever and shortness of breath for the previous four days on the mainland. He had recently had pneumonia, which he self-treated with antibiotics. Dr. Chow called in Dr. Wu Chun-wah, a consultant, who reassessed Dr. Liu. Somehow the question of the mainland outbreak of atypical pneumonia must have hung in the air, because according to Wu, Liu added that "he had already recovered and was not suffering 'that kind of thing.'"

"It was our understanding," Wu testified later, "that the patient was telling us that he was not suffering the type of atypical pneumonia recently reported in China." We don't know why he said that, but he would not be the last physician infected with SARS to underestimate the degree to which he was infected, or the outcome of traveling among the public.

Wu examined Liu, and the signs were not good: through the stethoscope he heard crackling sounds in both of Liu's lungs, and his chest X-rays revealed a "ground-glass appearance," both of which strongly suggested pneumonia. Suspecting as much, he admitted Liu to the intensive care unit.

Kwong Wah hospital, and everyone who worked there, were extremely fortunate. At the time Dr. Liu was admitted, the working party on community-acquired pneumonia had just recommended a higher level of infection control, and there just happened to be a spare bed in the isolation ward within the Intensive Care Unit (ICU). The admitting physician happened to be on good terms with the head of the ICU, and though neither of them had the slightest notion how important this decision would be, they decided to use the bed for Dr. Liu.

"We were so lucky," said Dr. Andrew Yip, head of surgery at Kwong Wah. If Liu had been placed in a general ward, as might well have been the case if the ICU had been full, then Kwong Wah might have gone through what the French Hospital in Viet Nam was about to undergo.

Even so, Liu's visit to Kwong Wah resulted in one infection—a registered nurse who attended a patient in the cubicle next to Liu's when he was in the emergency room. She was admitted to the hospital six days later, recovered, and was only later identified as a SARS case.

Two more pieces of luck followed in quick succession. As it happened, Kwong Wah was a sister hospital to the First Affiliated Hospital of Sun Yat-Sen at the University in Guangzhou, and the two held yearly joint symposia. The Medical Superintendent had become a good friend of Yip's, and this personal contact would provide a vital hole in the curtain of silence that ran along the Hong Kong/Guangdong border. He called to say that Liu was one of his own hospital's physicians and, more importantly, to tell Yip that in treating Liu, Yip might be dealing with an infectious disease. He warned Yip to raise the level of vigilance and infection control at Kwong Wah.

The other piece of luck was that Yip had been a classmate of Professor KY Yuen of the University of Hong Kong, one of the top microbiologists in the province. The two were close friends, and Yip called Yuen to talk the case over.

"He called me up," Yuen said, "and said, 'KY, something is wrong.'" He told Yuen that a professor from the Guangzhou Medical University was in his hospital with some kind of atypical pneumonia, perhaps connected to what was happening across the border.

Yuen himself was sick that day with flu, so he asked Dr. Ho Pak-Leung, a microbiologist, and Dr. Kenneth Tsang Wah-Tak, a respiratory specialist, to visit Kwong Wah Hospital in his place. Both wore highly protective gear, including disposable gowns, N95 masks, and gloves.

Ho came back and reported that Liu was indeed very ill, apparently with a viral pneumonia, and Yuen recommended Ribavirin, a broad-spectrum anti-viral medication.

While this was taking place in Hong Kong, a team of experts from the WHO Global Outbreak Alert and Response Network (GOARN) arrived in Beijing on February 23, hoping to make the short journey east to Guangdong to investigate the mysterious pneumonia outbreak, but they were denied permission to do so.

The next day, according to newspaper accounts, Dr. Watt Chi-Leung, director of the ICU at Kwong Wah, was surprised to hear that

Professor Liu had visitors: three senior doctors from Zhongshan University in Guangzhou. He arranged for them to discuss Liu's condition with a senior physician, and see their colleague from behind a glass window.

"They told us they did not know what caused the disease and they kept asking us about our findings," Watt said. "They were very anxious to find out whether we had identified the virus which caused the disease. They collected a photocopy of our medical report on the patient and left the hospital. We were unable to find them afterwards."

He said the hospital had kept no official record of this mysterious visit, but believed one of the doctors was the head of Zhongshan University Hospital.

When he was feeling better, Dr. Yuen went to see the patient for himself. "He was already very sick: intubated, 100% oxygen, both lungs white-out," said Yuen. In plain terms, Liu needed to have a tube down his windpipe, connected to a ventilator providing a high level of oxygen, and his lungs on an X-ray showed a severe degree of infection. The medical team decided to try intravenous immunoglobulin and steroids.

"Unfortunately by the time he was admitted he had been ill for more than six days. By the time I saw him, it was around day eight. He didn't make it."

* * *

It would be some time before it was known that Professor Liu was the index (i.e., first) SARS case in the outbreaks that followed in Viet Nam, Hong Kong, and Singapore. As late as March 21, Science was reporting that the first known case was one of the guests infected at the Metropole I'll call Jimmy Ho, who carried the virus to Viet Nam. Since then, though, Professor Liu has received that dubious distinction. In effect, he was demonized just by how he has been described: the person who caused the global SARS outbreak.

Yet it's also possible to look at his contribution to the events of 2002-2003 in a very different way. By taking the virus outside China, he triggered what might be thought of as the world's immune response. At least 8,098 people would contract the disease and at least 774 would die; on the other hand, the world would be given the opportunity to learn a great deal and potentially strengthen its ability to contain SARS in particular and infectious disease in general.

If he had stayed in China, it's possible the outbreak would have been far longer, and far worse. China might have delayed opening its doors to international help for much longer. The virus might have spread to rural areas where it would have overwhelmed the sparse health care facilities and personnel, and set up a more permanent human reservoir. There was also a very real and unfortunate likelihood that unless the First World felt threatened, it would have allowed China to go on dealing with its own problems, under the mistaken belief that an infectious disease would stay in its own backyard. Had the virus not reached Hong Kong and the world, the outcome might have been far more serious in the long run.

Professor Liu, then, might be the person who simultaneously delivered SARS to the world and delivered the world from SARS.

Chapter 7.

The Outbreak Spreads

On Wednesday, February 26, as Professor Liu was declining at an alarming rate, a middle-aged Chinese-American businessman we'll call Jimmy Ho was admitted to the French Hospital in Hanoi with a 3-day history of respiratory symptoms.

"It was a mystery," said Pascale Brudon, the WHO Country Representative in Hanoi, speaking over the phone from Viet Nam in French-accented English. "Myself, I first really learned about it on the third of March. On Friday, which was the last day of February, my colleague Dr. [Carlo] Urbani was called by the French Hospital in Hanoi because they were worried about this American patient and wanted some information about the avian flu.

"We knew there were cases of avian flu in Hong Kong. We also knew there was something going on in China, but we knew very little about it. The French Hospital had this patient coming from Hong Kong and mainland China. He was hospitalized on the 26th of February, and they called us on the 28th, worried about avian flu. Carlo went into the hospital over the weekend and again on Monday.

"The situation became worrying quite quickly because already on Wednesday seven health workers were sick. It was on Wednesday we were convinced that we had a major public health problem.

"Of course, we didn't know what it was. We knew it was not avian flu because at the very beginning of the week Carlo took samples and sent them to Hong Kong and Japan. He was a very good clinician, though, and even without the results of the tests he was sure it was not avian flu."

This single paragraph illustrates the enormous importance of the WHO Country Offices. A small hospital in a relatively small and not very affluent country was able to call in someone with international experience in infectious diseases, who knew how important it was to act quickly, and had the initiative, the experience, and the means to send specimens to laboratories of international quality. Next, he had the professional stature to persuade the hospital immediately to raise its standards of infection control and the national government to take the situation seriously and act promptly. Comparing the first few days' events in Viet Nam with the curtain-raising events elsewhere illustrates both how fortunate Viet Nam was, and how valuable a consultative role the WHO was able to take.

Sure enough, the labs in the WHO influenza network agreed with Urbani: it was not avian flu, and it was not any known respiratory illness. The red flag went up: a new disease was suspected, the WHO issued an advisory beginning "Since mid February, WHO has been actively working to confirm reports of outbreaks of a severe form of pneumonia in Viet Nam, Hong Kong Special Administrative Region (SAR), China, and Guangdong province in China," which went on to summarize what little was known at the time. Finally, the tracking process began in earnest. This was all Urbani's doing, and without his presence in Hanoi, the level of global awareness would probably have remained low for several more crucial days. For the WHO, at least for the next few weeks, the starting point of SARS was Hanoi.

Meanwhile, the situation in the French Hospital was deteriorating quickly.

"Then we began to be very worried, because more and more people were [falling] sick," Brudon continued. "We informed the government, of course, and in the beginning as it was in a private hospital, they didn't take it very seriously.

"[Starting Wednesday], Carlo tried to raise the level of infection control in the hospital. He tried to persuade them to separate the patients with infectious disease from the others. On Thursday I sent a letter to the government to explain all that, and also to the hospital to tell them they should reinforce their infection measures, and on Friday we asked for technical support from outside."

During these hectic few days, the WHO Country Office was in constant contact with headquarters and with its regional office in the Western Pacific (WPRO) in the Philippines. "At the beginning everyone was very worried about this famous influenza pandemic which now is the new subject of the year," Brudon said sardonically, "but when we discovered it was not [influenza], there were worries because it was obviously something serious, so we were communicating all the time with Geneva and with Manila."

Urbani was 46, a good candidate for the embodiment of the public health physician. Even as a student, he organized groups to take the handicapped on countryside picnics. As a family doctor, he took his vacations in Africa, traveling with a backpack full of medicine. As he became increasingly interested in tropical medicine he gravitated toward parasitology: he was an expert in Schistosoma mekongi in Vietnam, in the food-borne nematodes and trematodes of Laos and Cambodia, and the hookworms of the Maldives. Rather than becoming a pure researcher, though, he remained committed to public health. In Italy, he pushed Medecins Sans Frontieres into working with the poorest of the poor, with Gypsies in Rome and with African and Albanian boat people who were landing in Sicily and Calabria.

"Carlo always wanted to join WHO," Brudon said. "It was one of his wishes in life to be a doctor who served the world." He had already worked for WHO in Cambodia. "He was a very good parasitologist. Even when he was working in Italy as a doctor, he was working with our colleagues in Geneva. Then he got involved more and more in field work, partly with us and partly with other organizations. Then he was recruited for this post, and he was taking care of Laos, Cambodia, Viet Nam and also, for certain aspects of parasitic disease, China. He was the only clinician in the office at the time, and the one in charge of communicable disease. He had good relations with the people in the French Hospital—they trusted him, and they also trusted the WHO."

Herein, perhaps, lies a clue to the character of the Viet Nam outbreak: it was an outbreak with international dimensions. Jimmy Ho, the person bringing the virus into the country, went to the French Hospital, a small, two-floor hospital, staffed to a considerable degree by French doctors on short rotations, catering largely to the international community and to some wealthier Vietnamese. The French Hospital was in some ways the counterpart of the Metropole in Hong Kong: if the Metropole was a gateway to the world, the French Hospital was an international port of entry.

Brudon hypothesizes that if the carrier of the virus had been admitted to a large hospital catering primarily to Vietnamese, it's possible that the hospital would not have thought to contact the WHO so quickly. It's also very possible that the outbreak would have been worse because SARS had spread most rapidly within large hospitals with open admission or emergency areas, and substantial numbers of health care workers,patients, and visitors circulating around the corridors—less confinement in general for the virus.

Brudon agreed: "That's why in Hanoi, [SARS] was not a disaster for the health services. It was very difficult for the French Hospital, but Jimmy Ho came into the hospital quite quickly so he didn't pass the virus on to many people [beforehand]. I think he passed it to one or two people, but they were discharged very quickly-and then he was inside the hospital. The staff of the hospital, even the ones who were not sick, stayed in the hospital because they didn't want to put their families in danger. So the virus remained inside."

In East Africa, when someone in a small, remote village falls sick with Ebola hemorrhagic fever, his family practices a kind of rough-and-ready infection control: they shut him in the family hut with food and water, and leave him inside for several days. He may die, or he may recover, but that is out of their hands anyway, as there is no treatment for Ebola. The one thing he won't do either way is to infect anyone else.

The French Hospital was all but sealed off, and with the exception of the errant physicians, the virus did, on the whole, remain inside. Modern medical ethics, though, are not as brutal as those in Ebola-struck villages: instead of leaving the sick alone to recover or die, we try our best to make them better, or at least make them comfortable. We go into the hut.

Urbani's determination to investigate the cause of the illness and advise on infection control would prove fatal. On March 11, already feeling ill, he flew from Hanoi to Bangkok to give a presentation on tropical diseases. When the plane landed, a friend was there to meet him, but Urbani waved him back and the two sat in chairs eight feet apart until an ambulance arrived 90 minutes later, its frightened attendants having stopped for protective gear. He was taken to hospital, where an infection-proof isolation room had been hastily rigged up, with double panes of glass and fans to create negative air pressure so when a door was opened, air would flow in instead of out.

Over the next few days, he grew steadily weaker, and could breathe only through a respirator. In a conscious moment, he said he wanted his lung tissue saved for science.

Dr. Carlo Urbani died on March 29.

* * *

On March 1, 1,365 miles away in Singapore, a 26-year-old former flight attendant we'll call Elaine Lim was admitted to Tan Tock Seng Hospital in Singapore with respiratory symptoms. Five days later, she was in the hospital's intensive care unit. Meanwhile, the infection had spread to include her parents, her grandmother, and nearly twenty other people, and an infectious disease consultant named Dr. Lee Cheng Chuan was informing the Health Ministry about a rare infection that didn't respond to the usual antibiotics.

Lee knew that Lim had just returned from Hong Kong with a friend who was also showing similar symptoms; news was coming in of a third woman, also back from Hong Kong, and also in Tan Tock Seng, with this strange atypical pneumonia. On March 10, a nurse at the hospital fell sick and was admitted on the same day as Lim's mother. Two days later, another nurse started showing the same symptoms.

At first, doctors suspected dengue fever—or perhaps, given the Hong Kong connection, it was avian influenza. By the time authorities made the connection back through the Metropole to the Chinese outbreak of atypical pneumonia, they realized that as many as 1,500 people might already be infected.

Lim survived, but the first person to die of SARS in Singapore was her father. The second was her pastor, who had come to visit her.

* * *

On March 15, a 72-year-old man, who had been visiting a relative in the Prince of Wales Hospital in Hong Kong, flew to Beijing on China Air Flight 112. He had already begun to develop SARS symptoms, but when he arrived in Beijing the symptoms were not recognized: he was evaluated at one hospital but sent home. The next day, his family took him to the emergency department of a second Beijing hospital, where he had to be resuscitated before being admitted. He died there on March 20, by which time he had infected at least 59 people, including three of his immediate family, six of the seven health-care workers who resuscitated him in the emergency room, one other health care worker, and other patients and their contacts. The virus also seems to have been passed on to others on Flight 112, leading to subsequent cases in Taiwan and Inner Mongolia.

* * *

By this time the virus had also stolen into Canada, infecting a 78-year-old woman visiting family in Hong Kong: she stayed at the Metropole only because the travel package that she bought included three nights' stay at the Metropole. She returned to Canada, developed a confusing range of symptoms, and died at home without ever being admitted to a hospital. She had lived with an extended family that consisted of her husband, a daughter, two sons, a son-in-law, and a grandchild. All but one contracted the infection before the outbreak reached the attention of the medical authorities.

"It started on March 9th," recalled Dr. Barbara Yaffe, at the time the acting Medical Officer of Health for the city of Toronto. Yaffe is an emphatic and spirited woman with retro-hip rectangular glasses and a penchant for speaking her mind. "I was on call; it was a Sunday. The manager on call had a call from Scarborough Grace Hospital with what they thought was possibly several cases of tuberculosis. The manager called me and I said, 'Isolate them and refer it to the TB unit in the morning.'

"The TB team investigated, and it was coming back negative for TB. By the middle of the week, it started to look more serious. We had a 43-year-old man who was very sick—he was in [the] ICU and in fact died. Then we found out his mother had died the previous week. She supposedly had died of a heart attack at home. There was no autopsy done, but she had just been in Hong Kong. Then the World Health Organization alert came out [on March 12] about atypical pneumonia. We started to put it all together. Several other members of the family were getting very ill very quickly. By the evening of March 13th we were having an emergency teleconference with the province. By Friday we realized, 'We really have a big problem here.'

"I was the acting medical officer of health. The medical officer of health was on holiday—good timing on her part!—and I had to do a press conference that Friday night, March 14th, with the Ministry of Health and a local infectious disease specialist to say that we had a cluster of very severe atypical pneumonia in a family, one of whom had just come back from Hong Kong.

"That Friday we mobilized all the staff we could for the next day to set up a hotline. Of course, it happened on a Friday, as usual. It hit the front pages of all our major papers and all the news outlets that night and Saturday—and it just kind of went on from there. This took over our lives until the end of June.

"I don't think any of us had time to think through any of it. It went from one crazy thing to the next. Instead of getting better, it kept getting worse. Myself, I wished I had time to sit back and really look at the data and think through it as a group, and do the planning, but we just didn't have the time. We were desperate. We were asking for help. We asked for epidemiologists from Health Canada. They sent a small number, and then they were taken away by the province. We were just desperate. We were bringing in staff who normally don't do this kind of work.

We didn't have policies and procedures like you have on diseases you know about. We didn't know anything. We didn't know what disease we were dealing with, we didn't know how it was transmitted, we didn't know its incubation period. All we knew was that people were coming down with this thing, it was pretty bad, and it was spreading."

* * *

On March 10, the management of the Prince of Wales Hospital, a 1,200-bed teaching hospital in the New Territories area of Hong Kong, was notified that seven doctors and four nurses had all gone on sick leave at the same time—and all of them worked in Ward 8A.

The ward was immediately closed to visitors and new patients while the hospital tried to work out what was going on. The following day the number of staff on sick leave from Ward 8A was up to 14, even though the patients in the ward didn't seem to show signs of any unusual illness. By late evening, more staff were falling sick, including three cardiothoracic surgeons who had visited the ward the previous week. When the hospital management required all health care staff currently on sick leave—now up to 50—to get a checkup, no fewer than 23 had fevers and/or signs of pneumonia on X-ray, and were immediately isolated in the observation ward of the accident and emergency department, which had been hurriedly cleared to make room.

(A side note: SARS was ruthlessly exposing health care weaknesses wherever it went, but the Prince of Wales experience illustrated an area that is still poorly recognized—occupational health surveillance among health care workers. Many nurses and some doctors work in more than one hospital or clinic, and if someone is out sick often nobody knows why. British Columbia is setting up an occupational health surveillance system to track who is out sick and why—which will give an early warning of hospital-centered infectious disease. While this could help track recurring injuries and design safer hospitals, such thinking is still largely in the pre-implementation phase.)

Dr. David Hui, a pulmonary specialist at the Prince of Wales Hospital, described the events a year and a day after the outbreak began.

"Between the 8th and the 10th of March 2003 there were more and more people from Ward 8A having a febrile illness [i.e., an illness with fever] that mimicked flu. On the 11th of March, 50 colleagues called in sick. So we called an emergency clinic on the 11th of March at 8 p.m. to find out what was going on. These people were all red and hot and very tired-looking. We performed X-rays, we did physical examinations, blood tests, and out of the fifty colleagues that we screened, 8 of them had very obvious pneumonia on X-ray. I was responsible for seeing all the X-rays from all these patients. And the other patients were also quite unwell, so we worked from 8 p.m. until midnight, and then we decided to admit 23 colleagues to our hospital for observation.

"We had an urgent department meeting to discuss what to do, where to place these colleagues, and we didn't finish until 1:30 in the morning and then the next day we all returned to work at 7 a.m. and from then on, every day we admitted 20 to 30 new cases.

"In the two weeks after the onset of the outbreak we admitted 156 patients and by the end of the epidemic we were up to 347 just within the Prince of Wales. So it was a major outbreak.

"It was terrible. Many of the patients were my colleagues and 40% of my department of medicine members were infected. Because [so many] were down, we had to divide the remaining members into 'dirty' teams and 'clean' teams. The dirty team members only looked after the atypical pneumonia cases, whereas the clean team members would continue looking after the non-SARS patients.

"At the beginning we had no idea what it was. It was all mysterious. The term SARS was only coined on the fifteenth of March and the coronavirus was only identified on the 22nd. So in the first couple of weeks it was just like fighting in the dark."

Residents living near the Prince of Wales hospital in the district of Sha Tin began clearing pharmacy shelves of masks, antibiotics, and Chinese remedies. One pharmacy owner told the South China Morning Post that he had sold five dozen masks in one morning.

A salesman outside the hospital handed out fliers for air purifiers, whose copy, in Chinese, read: "Atypical pneumonia—Hong Kong, Guangzhou, and Viet Nam already plagued. Use Bionaire air-purifiers to lower the risk of infection. Special offer as low as $441, effective until 28th of April—but date may be extended as long as the flu attack continues."

The three models of purifier cost roughly between US$80 and $190. Hospital staff and patients qualified for a 25 per cent reduction.

* * *

News of all of these events was passed on to the WHO in Geneva, which in addition to monitoring and discussing the spreading outbreak was about to get a wake-up call of a particularly literal kind.

Chapter 8.

Where the Hell is This Guy?

The WHO headquarters in Geneva consists of a group of buildings set in the stately parkland up on a hill near the United Nations building, the whole area giving the impression that all the world's troubles can be sorted out in good time by intelligent discussion among reasonable people.

The flagship building within the WHO complex is massive and graceful, something between an ocean liner and a battleship, fluttering the flags of a hundred nations. Next to it, Batiment M, home to the Communicable Disease Surveillance and Response Department (CDS), looks like an organic egg carton.

It's a maxim of the building that nobody ever sees the CDS people-they're always off somewhere coping with an outbreak of something-but the department still seems absurdly overcrowded. The offices are not spacious, so most of the doors are usually open. The view of the narrow corridor reveals a steady thoroughfare of well-heeled flooring lined with filing cabinets, walls decorated with photos of cultures of meningitis, pneumonia, and influenza on blood-red circular agar plates, and a prominent picture of a person lying on his side, with instructions on how to deliver a lumbar puncture.

Batiment M gives a vivid illustration of what the WHO can do well, and what it can't. In talking to a variety of people who had little direct knowledge of the WHO, it became clear that to many it seemed like a battleship: a weighty entity that might be dispatched to steam at deliberate speed around the globe and arrive in some remote port to quell a local disturbance—and as such, a creature of the imperial era, to be resented as often as admired.

Even if this may have been true once, the WHO was changing, and nothing changed it more urgently than the phone call that woke Mike Ryan, the coordinator of GOARN, at 2:00 a.m. on March 15th, 2003.

"That was the seminal week in the whole response, because up 'til then we had kind of this phoney war where we had the avian flu cases from Fujian, and then we had the Vietnam situation—Carlo [Urbani] had reported that, and we had just sent a team to the field. By the 12th we had decided, 'This is not influenza, but we don't know what it is,' so we put out that initial alert, warning people about atypical pneumonia of unknown cause. But it wasn't a global alert saying, 'Oh, my God, watch out!' It was really a notification to clinicians to watch out that there clearly was a pneumonia-like illness—it doesn't appear to be influenza, and it's caused a cluster [of infections] in a health care setting. And it was the cluster in that health care setting that really sparked us to put that initial alert out.

"Between that day—which was a Wednesday—and that Friday, Canada lit up, Hong Kong lit up, Singapore too... we started to see little explosions of this atypical pneumonia all over the place in health care settings, which in itself was very worrying.

"Friday night we were contemplating the whole thing. Was the initial alert strong enough? Had we hit the right tone, you know? Trying to get teams to go to Hong Kong, teams to go everywhere. So we were definitely going to come in on Saturday," he chuckled. "It was going to be a normal business day! Clearly, all of us went home on Friday thinking, 'This situation is changing.'

"That night, then, was the first time we moved into the real-time element. Up to then we were getting the reports from the countries slightly retrospectively: 'We've had cases today, or yesterday... But this was the first time we were talking about a real-time event."

"About two or three o'clock in the morning I got a call from Prof. Chiu in the Singapore Health Office. I was at home asleep, but I was getting up a lot of nights. During that period there was no such thing as sleep. We were getting one hour of sleep, then on the phone for two and on the email for three. It wasn't a big thing to be woken up. Many, many times, with teams in the field you get woken up in the middle of the night.

"So it was Prof. Chiu saying, basically, 'Bit of a situation here. One of our clinicians, who went to a conference in New York, got sick.'

"'Oh, I say. 'Where is he? What hospital?'

"'Well,' he says, 'it's not as simple as that. He went to the hospital, had an X-ray, and didn't phone us.' He'd obviously phoned colleagues or family members to say he was sick, he'd had an X-ray and he was coming home.

"'Well, certainly, you should have him isolated in New York.'

"'It's not as simple as that. He's got on an airplane and we think he's going to Heathrow.

"I said, "Singapore Airlines. Fine. Do you have the flight number?'

"'No, we just think he's on the flight. There aren't that many Singapore Airlines flights.'

"So I immediately picked up the phone and got Angus Nichol out of bed. He's the head of the Communicable Disease Surveillance Centre in England. I said 'Angus! Good mornin'! Here's the deal. . . .'

"He went, 'Oh, my God. Well, I'd better get on to that.'"

Nichol rang the medical office at Heathrow, but more bad news was on its way.

"About twenty minutes later, half an hour later, I got a call back from Angus, saying, `This guy is not on this flight. In fact, we don't even think there is such a flight. We've checked all the other airlines, and there's nobody of this name.'

"So I'm thinking, Where the hell is this guy?"

The SARS ante was rising. The WHO already knew that people with the atypical pneumonia were flying all over the world, taking it with them, but this was the first time that they knew of a case as it was happening, and might be able to do something about it.

"So I called back Singapore and said, 'He's not on that flight.' It's Saturday afternoon there, so everything's closed. They said, 'We'll try and check with the airline, and with the company that arranged his travel to the medical conference to see what his itinerary was.' They went around trying to contact family members, came back and said, 'Yep, you're right, he's not on the flight to London.'

"So I'm thinking, 'Good, he's in New York.'

"[Then they said], 'No, he's on a flight to Frankfurt. And the flight's already left.'

"So I'm counting [time zones] on my fingers, six minus five—where is he now? Somewhere over the Azores or wherever, you know?"

Ryan knew that the physician was already showing symptoms of the disease—why else would he go for an X-ray? Now he found out that the victim was traveling with his pregnant wife and his mother-in-law: every new piece of information seemed to ratchet up the tension.

Ryan called the German authorities, who moved quickly.

"So the poor man—when the airplane arrived in Frankfurt it was taken off to the side, these guys in space suits came running in and grabbed these three people, and everyone else on the plane [another

155 passengers] was held. Should they all be put in quarantine or should they not? You're trying to develop policy. So [the Germans] implemented their standard procedures, which were totally adequate. The doctor from Singapore was isolated. Everyone was interviewed and they looked at the high-risk contacts [who had been sitting near the Singapore party] and asked them to remain for active follow-up. All the contact details for all the people on the plane were taken, and everyone else was allowed to go home. That was that.

"So I arrived," Ryan chuckled, "pale as a sheet on Saturday morning. That incident and other incidents—everyone had the sense that things had really gone pear-shaped. You only had to walk in the door. There was a real sense of, well, the curtain's gone up now! This is it. Full-court press.

"That morning we really decided, look, we've documented international transfer of the disease to different countries, we've seen symptomatic health workers getting on planes, potentially exposing hundreds of people. We clearly have to get a much stronger message out to the world.

"We started to stitch together a press release to go with that, but we were also working on all kinds of documentation: surveillance definitions, definitions of the disease, all of that. It was a new disease, and we had to go out to the world not only with 'Here's a new disease,' but 'Here's how you recognize it, here's how you manage it."

Once the press release was out, the team looked at each other and realized they needed to give the disease a name.

They were keen to avoid the tradition of naming an illness by its country or region of origin (Asian flu, Hong Kong flu) so as not to start a process of blame.

"Hanoi Syndrome, or whatever! No, no. Well, first of all it had to be a syndrome because we didn't know what it was, and we had to get across the severity of it and the acuteness of it, and try to get across in the name some indication of what it was. The last thing we wanted was to put out an alert for everyone walking down the street in any country in the world to think, 'Oh my God, that person has got that new disease. People don't read the case definition, so we tried to incorporate into the name an indication of the case definition: Severe. Acute. Respiratory. Syndrome. To give the idea that this is not the normal thing you see walking down the streets. A worrying message but reassuring at the same time!" he chuckled.

The message, couched in the deliberate, restrained language of the WHO, ran in its entirety as follows:

World Health Organization issues emergency travel advisory

15 March 2003

15 March 2003 | GENEVA—During the past week, WHO has received reports of more than 150 new suspected cases of Severe Acute Respiratory Syndrome (SARS), an atypical pneumonia for which cause has not yet been determined. Reports to date have been received from Canada, China, Hong Kong Special Administrative Region of China, Indonesia, Philippines, Singapore, Thailand, and Viet Nam. Early today, an ill passenger and companions who traveled from New York, United States, and who landed in Frankfurt, Germany were removed from their flight and taken to hospital isolation.

Due to the spread of SARS to several countries in a short period of time, the World Health Organization today has issued emergency guidance for travelers and airlines.

"This syndrome, SARS, is now a worldwide health threat," said Dr. Gro Harlem Brundtland, Director General of the World Health Organization. "The world needs to work together to find its cause, cure the sick, and stop its spread."

There is presently no recommendation for people to restrict travel to any destination. However in response to enquiries from governments, airlines, physicians and travelers, WHO is now offering guidance for travelers, airline crew and airlines. The exact nature of the infection is still under investigation and this guidance is based on the early information available to WHO.

TRAVELLERS INCLUDING AIRLINE CREW: All travellers should be aware of main symptoms and signs of SARS which include:

high fever (>38(C)

one or more respiratory symptoms including cough, shortness of breath, difficulty breathing

AND one or more of the following:

close contact with a person who has been diagnosed with SARS

recent history of travel to areas reporting cases of SARS.

In the unlikely event of a traveller experiencing this combination of symptoms they should seek medical attention and ensure that information about their recent travel is passed on to the health care staff. Any traveller who develops these symptoms is advised not to undertake further travel until they have recovered.

AIRLINES: Should a passenger or crew member who meets the criteria above travel on a flight, the aircraft should alert the destination airport. On arrival the sick passenger should be referred to airport health authorities for assessment and management. The aircraft passengers and crew should be informed of the person's status as a suspect case of SARS. The passengers and crew should provide all contact details for the subsequent 14 days to the airport health authorities. There are currently no indications to restrict the onward travel of healthy passengers, but all passengers and crew should be advised to seek medical attention if they develop the symptoms highlighted above. There is currently no indication to provide passengers and crew with any medication or investigation unless they become ill.

In the absence of specific information regarding the nature of the organism causing this illness, specific measures to be applied to the aircraft cannot be recommended. As a general precaution the aircraft may be disinfected in the manner described in the WHO Guide to Hygiene and Sanitation in Aviation.

* * *

As more information has become available, WHO-recommended SARS case definitions have been revised as follows:

Suspect Case

A person presenting after 1 February 2003 with history of:
* high fever (>38(C)
AND
* one or more respiratory symptoms including cough, shortness of breath, difficulty breathing
* close contact1 with a person who has been diagnosed with SARS
* recent history of travel to areas reporting cases of SARS

Probable Case

A suspect case with chest X-ray findings of pneumonia or Respiratory Distress Syndrome

OR

A person with an unexplained respiratory illness resulting in death, with an autopsy examination demonstrating the pathology of Respiratory Distress Syndrome without an identifiable cause.

Comments

In addition to fever and respiratory symptoms, SARS may be associated with other symptoms including: headache, muscular stiffness, loss of appetite, malaise, confusion, rash, and diarrhea.

* * *

Until more is known about the cause of these outbreaks, WHO recommends that patients with SARS be isolated with barrier nursing techniques and treated as clinically indicated. At the same time, WHO recommends that any suspect cases be reported to national health authorities.

WHO is in close communication with all national authorities and has also offered epidemiological, laboratory and clinical support. WHO is working with national authorities to ensure appropriate investigation, reporting and containment of these outbreaks.

*Close contact means having cared for, having lived with, or having had direct contact with respiratory secretions and body fluids of a person with SARS.

For more information contact:

Dick Thompson—Communication Officer Communicable Disease Prevention, Control and Eradication WHO, Geneva Telephone: (+41 22) 791 26 84 Email: thompsond@who.int

---

The press release itself represented a sea-change in the way the WHO worked: it was an attempt to emerge from the labyrinthine corridors of global bureaucracy and give up a certain amount of control in order to deal with a disease outbreak in real time—that is, to move at the same rate as the disease.

"Unlike a normal public health challenge," Ryan explained, "[this was] an emergent policy thing. Where you go through the normal route—WHO sends documents to the Ministry, the Ministry passes them on and they cascade down—we didn't at that time have a fool-proof method of communicating with health ministries, and even if we did, it was the weekend. The fact was, if an individual got off a plane and walked into an emergency room, how long would it take for the cascade of warning to work? So, we basically used the media to get the message out. And it was amazing the number of clinicians [who] would come up to me over the last year at conferences and say, `D'you know, I was driving to work on the Saturday morning,' or `I was having my coffee and I heard that thing... ' It was on every news wire and every broadcast within four hours of the press release coming out. That was what got the information to the health workers at the front end—at that was what was important, because they were the ones who were at risk."

A few notes about the text of the advisory:

• These were recommendations, not orders. Even when the advisory said, "the aircraft should alert the destination airport . . . the sick passenger should be referred to airport health authorities...aircraft passengers and crew should be informed of the person's status as a suspect case of SARS," these remained pieces of advice. The WHO has no authority over governments or airlines.

• The advisory did not include any travel restrictions, with the exception of people who might actually have SARS. Individual governments were not so restrained: almost at once, a bewildering and contradictory series of restrictions and bans would be issued, raising the general level of confusion and anxiety.

• The phrase "As more information has become available" embodied the rolling nature of these advisories. Under the rapidly-changing circumstances at the beginning of any outbreak of infectious disease, as Mike Ryan put it, "That was the real challenge for the WHO: how do you generate real-time policy that's going to have major impact on travel, trade and public health systems using data from multiple sources that isn't perfect?"

In other words: Watch this space. The WHO's website received from 6 to 10 million hits per day during the peak months of the outbreak, from mid-March 2003 through the end of May that year, that number being highest when they issued or removed travel recommendations. At the beginning of the outbreak, the site issued situation updates each day except Sundays; Saturday updates continued until June. Altogether, there were 96 daily situation updates, with the last issued on July 5 with the welcome announcement that all known chains to human-to-human transmission had been broken.

• The "barrier nursing techniques" recommended by the WHO are precautions designed to prevent the health care staff catching whatever is infecting the patient. Across the world, different countries and different health care establishments would respond to this recommendation with varying degrees of caution. Some would end up wearing every piece of personal protective equipment (PPE) they could lay their hands on; others would take the recommendation lightly, to their cost.

• The name SARS may seem bland enough, but in fact it caused an immediate problem. There was a 12-day delay in adding SARS to the list of diseases for which people could be forced into quarantine because Hong Kong's health chief was opposed to calling the illness SARS and had doubts about its definition. Specifically, Hong Kong's Secretary for Health, Welfare and Food, Yeoh Eng-kiong, was worried that the name was ambiguous and misleading—not in terms of health, but politics. Hong Kong, since being returned to China from British rule in 1999, is technically called the Hong Kong Special Administrative Region, or SAR—entirely too close for comfort to the plural-sounding SARS. The steering committee chaired by Chief Executive Tung Chee-hwa dickered over the name, leading to a twelve-day delay in adding SARS to the list of quarantinable diseases as well as in implementing prevention measures such as designated medical centers for SARS patients, school closures, and border controls.

• In one respect, the WHO may have miscalculated—or perhaps this was the result of giving up some of its control over information by passing it over to the world media. In all the news articles that burst out all over the world like a flock of homing pigeons being released from their cages, the most common adjective is "unprecedented." The perception was that WHO had never taken this step before, therefore it must be a sign of the utmost urgency and danger. In fact, the step was unprecedented because the WHO was changing. It had never had the capacity to mobilize a worldwide response to a worldwide infectious disease before, so it had never assumed that role. GOARN was still new, and it had been tested only in local or regional outbreaks. Major changes were taking place in an international organization whose role was probably never especially clear, and no matter how many press releases the WHO had sent out to announce these changes, the news had not gripped the imagination of the international press corps or the public. The unprecedented step was actually very good news, because it was a sign that a new concerted global system was moving into action exactly as it had been designed.

If people misread the WHO release to some extent, perhaps it was because they saw the WHO not as a rapid response force but as a battleship: slow, reliable, heavy, impregnable. They were used to it being massive, perhaps authoritative, but definitely cautious. This was a different paradigm. This was like the Oxford English Dictionary publishing a handbook of slang: its very up-to-dateness, the currency of its language and information, was going to be something of a shock.

* * *

The press release of March 15 was just a sign that Batiment M was moving into high gear. The CDR team worked in two areas: (1) technical coordination and response, and (2) policy management.

The two clearly overlap: there's no point in discussing the outbreak without making a policy to deal with it, and you can't make a policy without good information. And as with many aspects of the WHO operation, the key was linkage: how to make sure that coordination/response and policy actually did overlap.

This was the work of David Heymann and Guanael Rodier.

"They were the lynchpins," Ryan explained, "in turning technical advice and technical assessment into WHO policy—basically, the DG's decisions. David was not only the front man for the outbreak, but also at the front end of generating policy proposals. Guenael was in a similar role, but he also kept all the regional offices and ourselves talking to each other, holding teleconferences, making sure that WPRO [Western Pacific Regional Office] activity and WPRO policy was in line with our policy, and [coordinating] at the country level, keeping that constant communication."

These activities may sound tediously bureaucratic, but even spelling them out distorts the degree of pressure that everyone was working under. It's any bureaucrat's job to maintain a clear view of and control over his or her domain; it's not so common to be in a position where a lapse in communication or a brief difference in policy understanding might have immediate and fatal results. The WHO response was based on the need for both speed and consistency. Dithering—a bureaucrat's fallback position—was out of the question; letting each country come up with its own set of treatment guidelines and public health advisories would have been an invitation to uninformed judgments and global panic. Policy needed to interface with expert technical assessment, and vice versa, and it all had to happen at once.

Ryan was in overall charge of assessing and coordinating GOARN's response. "I [could be considered] the first level of technical coordination—coordinating the field operations, teams in the field, gathering surveillance information, production of guidelines and all of that."

Tom Grein and the operations team focused on the logistics of getting teams out into the field. "Mobilizing the GOARN mechanism, finding the money, getting people out into the field in twenty-four hours."

Even the process of tracking all the incoming information, sifting, sorting, and presenting the most vital statistics—a standard activity in Batiment M that takes place before the daily morning briefing-involved such a torrent of incoming information, rumor and questions that the team and the meeting had to split in two like an amoeba, with one squad trying to handle SARS while the other took on everything else that was wrong with the world.

Meanwhile, an equally complex and ambitious response was being run at the regional level out of the Western Pacific Regional Office (abbreviated to WPRO and pronounced "whip-row") by Hitoshi Oshitani, mobilizing troops and managing resources in the region, the main theater in the war against SARS. It was especially important to share duties between WPRO and Geneva. "If WPRO couldn't mobilize consultants because it was six in the evening, we would be in the next morning and we'd do it."

As information became policy, it turned into information again—and during SARS, that information was news. Within the press office, Mary Kay Kindhauser began the news cycle by running the WHO web, and Dick Thompson carried it on by answering questions for the hundreds of news stories that ran daily across the world. Thompson took so many phone calls at every hour of the day and night that he wore his hands-free phone set under his helmet so he could talk to the press while cycling to and from work.

As head of PR for the WHO, Thompson spent the entire outbreak trying to pass on accurate non-inflammatory information, all the while working with incomplete data. It was a constant quandary: if the WHO was cautious with its information, knowing that it was subject to change and also to misinterpretation, then the organization might be accused of hiding things from the public, and the vacuum created by the lack of information would be filled with speculation, each round more extreme than the actual facts. On the other hand, if the WHO went public with incomplete data and was immediately shown to have been wrong, the loss of public confidence could be catastrophic.

"You've got just specks of information," Thompson said, a hint of challenge in his voice. "What do you do with that information? Do you sit on it until it becomes a coherent whole? Do you give it out and let people make what they want with it, even if they're sometimes wrong? Somebody's got to look at these dots of information and say, 'Some of these dots are important, some aren't.' There's a lot you have to discount. There's a few strands that are important but you don't know how they're connected. And there are huge blank spaces—like China—where you know there should be information."

"What would you do?" he wonders aloud.

What the WHO could do, since the inception of GOARN, was to put out a call to experts all over the world, organize them into teams, and send them to countries that had asked for help. This was where the ecumenical nature of the WHO became very useful. A war was taking place in Iraq at the time, and the world was polarized along critical fault lines: Islamic and non-Islamic countries; countries that signed on for the war and countries that refused. SARS, by stark contrast, was a universal peril: nobody refused to help, and conversely, the WHO could send teams under the blue helmet, so to speak, without offending nationalist sentiments.

(Well, almost. Certain First World countries have never called on the WHO for help and would probably refuse to do so for fear of seeming as if they are above such charity. The distinction between this attitude and, say, China's early disinclination to ask for help is thinner than it might seem.)

The number of teams in the field changed from week to week—Viet Nam, Singapore, China, Hong Kong, Taiwan—as did the number of people.

Ryan continued, "In Viet Nam, there were probably twelve or fourteen people. Hong Kong went up to six or seven. China, at one point—must have been twenty. Depending on the needs, different personnel from different backgrounds, changing over time.

"In places like China, the team was [initially] focused very much on the surveillance aspect, getting samples, and then to supporting the clinical management of the cases. Then, there would have been animal experts in there trying to look at SARS.

"The initial response to most epidemics would be to look at what we suspect the disease to be. In the recent Nipah [virus] outbreak in Bangladesh, when we didn't know what that was in the beginning, but we thought it could be avian flu, because there were some reports of dead chickens. But, we also thought it could be Nipah—we'd had Nipah there before and it sounded clinically like Nipah—so we crafted a team that could cover both angles. A couple of ecologists, an epidemiologist, a clinician; someone with experience in clinical management of dangerous pathogens. Much more an investigation team: characterize the illness, take the samples. Not necessarily containment, because it's a small outbreak.

"Whereas if we go to an Ebola outbreak, our primary objective is containment, so it'll be logistics and clinical management and health education. In the Congo for Ebola, we had anthropologists in the first wave of the team because access to the community is the key thing, and in pygmy communities you don't get access. So we had French anthropologists with expertise in pygmy anthropology on the team, not lab people. But then when you've established containment you bring in the scientists. Countries control outbreaks, not WHO, but we can add very precise resources.

"I didn't realize until a few weeks ago that we had chainsaws in our outbreak response kit. To get into the field in Congo last time, they had to cut seventy trees down. They had to build a new road just to get to the outbreak site. That's the reality of working under those conditions, which are very different to, say, sending a team to Hong Kong."

One of the common experiences of those who fought SARS was that it began with a phone call and a sudden geographical dislocation.

"I was based in Fiji at the WHO office in Suva, the regional office for the south Pacific," said Rob Condon of the WHO. "I'd been there for eight days when I received an email from this office saying, 'Urgent. Urgent. Urgent. Travel details to China and all points North.

"In my innocence, I wasn't expecting to get this on my eighth day in Fiji, and I thought maybe they'd sent the email to the wrong person by mistake. So I rang up and said, 'I think this sounds important. You'd better find the right person quickly.' They said, 'No, no, no. You're the right person. We want you to jump on a plane and come up to Manila.'"

Manila turned out to be one of the two hubs of the entire operation.

"My main job here was coordinating the field teams, and the field outbreak response. In the region we've had a number of outbreaks, as everybody is aware. These were originally in Viet Nam and Hong Kong, when I arrived here, and then an outbreak appeared in Singapore very shortly after I arrived here, and subsequently the whole China situation had to be folded into our strategic approach in the region as well."

This was not a frantic, all-hands call, though. It was crucial to get the right people in the right places to meet the right needs at the right time. One common need was simply to get the torrent of data under control; and in order to do that in Singapore, GOARN plucked Dan Rosen, a data manager, from a hill station in Kenya.

"Typically, in an outbreak of this kind, when it starts you are usually using paper records or Excel spreadsheets, not a form of database. You really don't know what data you're collecting, what you need to do. That quickly becomes overwhelming and it needs to be really organized, but the people in the middle of the crisis have a lot of trouble doing that, so they bring someone like me and try to take a step back and organize things."

* * *

GOARN was already adept at mobilizing field teams; what was new about SARS was that GOARN mobilized non-field teams. "Virtual networks," Ryan said. "Not necessarily putting experts on a plane and giving them a backpack and saying, `See you in six weeks', but getting the best brains in the world around virtual tables and videoconferences and emails and secure websites and telephone conferences."

Three virtual networks were set up. One was Klaus Stohr's lab group, set up to investigate what Ryan called "the etiology of the disease. In other words, 'What the hell is it?'" One was a clinicians' group, run by Mark Salter in the United Kingdom. The third was an epidemiology-and-surveillance group led by Angela Merianos, on loan from Australia, that was culling the incoming information from different countries and trying to work out the incubation period, the rate of infection, trying to set up mathematical models that would predict best- and worse-case scenarios for the rate of spread.

These groups will be examined more closely in a later chapter. What's worth noting now is that this was yet another example of the Heymann Doctrine in action: In each case, the CDR was trying to spin connections like a spider between existing resources (people, labs, programs, equipment) rather than trying to run the outbreak itself. The trick was to take all the different experts working on SARS and bring their expertise together; and then to take the results of that collaboration and turn it into policy.

"That's what the whole SARS thing was about, for us: the meeting of David's attempts over the last seven, eight years with Guenael, myself and others, to generate a credible operational technical group that can actually deal with epidemics, linked into all the partners around the world—that scientific and operational platform—but to have the bravery to use that, to link into immediate policy decision-making, turning that information, where you've actually got people generating the case definition, and as you're generating it you're printing it into the update that's going onto the Web.

"That takes a certain amount of courage. That's where David was sublime. Because you're going to be wrong, and you're going to be criticized, because you're going to put out preliminary information based on what you know now, and that's not particularly instinctive for public health policy people. We like to be sure of ourselves. We tend to take the physician's approach rather than the surgeon's approach. I was trained as a surgeon," he laughed. "The old shoot-first-and-ask-questions-later. You're always trained, as a surgeon, that there should be a certain proportion of normal things you take out. If everything you take out is diseased, you've probably missed [something]."

"In other words," he went on, turning serious, "you have to have the instinct to intervene."

The SARS outbreak team then, though it had the full resources of the WHO on call, was nothing like a battleship/aircraft carrier. It consisted of barely a dozen people in managerial roles and another dozen in support roles, none of whom was a SARS expert—there was no such animal—and many of whom had other outbreaks or issues to contend with at the same time. Even while they were recruiting players from governments and health organizations to draft into the field, they were trying to work out how to pay their salaries. It was the first full-scale rollout for a new way of addressing global infectious disease, and nobody knew how well, or indeed if, it would work.

Chapter 9.

In the Hospitals

By the end of March 2003, SARS had completely changed the nature and character of hospitals.

Instead of places of healing, they had become places of infection and danger. Instead of doctors and nurses being just the caregivers, they also became the victims, and instead of being the ones who protected the public, they found themselves transmitting the virus and being treated like lepers. Hospital design turned out to be entirely unsuitable for coping with infectious disease, creating large open spaces where the virus could readily pass from one person to another, and lifesaving technologies turned out also to be spreading the virus more broadly and efficiently than it could spread itself.

Yet at the same time, hospitals were more essential than ever. The paradox stretched individual institutions and even whole health care systems almost to the snapping point, and radically changed people's understanding of how hospitals should be designed, built, and run.

As soon as SARS struck them, hospitals were transformed into places of confusion, uncertainty, and fear.

"I responded to the global outbreak and alert response network call for volunteers to go to Viet Nam even before we knew SARS existed," said Dr. Aileen Plant, Professor of International Health at Curtin University, Australia. "All we knew was that there was a respiratory illness happening there.

"I found a lot of ill patients, all in one hospital, the Hanoi French Hospital, at that stage. It's a little hospital, it's only got fifty-odd beds. About 200 people work there if you include the gardeners and the drivers and everybody, and forty of those people got ill with SARS. We can't imagine what it was like for doctors and nurses to first of all see their colleagues getting sick and then feeling the symptoms themselves and then seeing their colleagues die and not knowing whether they were going to live or die. All they knew was that it was something new and weird.

"That was undoubtedly the worst aspect of SARS, that human side that we can't imagine, you know. For a nurse, thinking, 'Will I go home tonight? Are my children going to catch this if I get it?' Or going home and finding that your family doesn't want you home. Or that nobody is coming to your restaurant any more because they might catch SARS. That's how people felt."

"The initial stages were difficult," said Dr. Brenda Ang of Tan Tock Seng Hospital in Singapore, "because people were very, very worried. People were saying, 'Can it be in the air conditioning? Can you get it by going to the canteen? We really didn't know at that time, so the first two weeks was probably quite crucial in the sense that we had to try and convince people that it was safe to work."

All the same, in most SARS-struck institutions it was the sense of common threat that created a common resolve. The crisis tore down the usual institutional barriers—between researchers and clinicians, between surgeons and physicians, and MDs and nurses.

"There was a general sense of fear, even among professionals," said Dr. Andrew Yip of Kwong Wah Hospital in Hong Kong. "The disease was so infectious, we were all in it together. The surgeons had to help out. It was all chaos. [The hospital] needed more beds, more space, more rooms. We cut our workload in half, postponed all non-essential surgeries—and that was a [nuisance] because we had to call every single patient who had an appointment and explain that we'd have to see them in a couple of months—and we gave two of our four wards to [SARS patients]."

The system was so overtaxed that surgeons were also needed to become general clinicians. "If we stuck to our turf, it wouldn't help anything." Yip called his staff together and they discussed the situation. The ICU needed staff—a high-risk and possibly fatal assignment. "It was like wartime. We drew lots as to who would go first. The surgeons with families would go into the hazardous areas last; those who were single would go first. At the worst time we had two surgeons working in the ICU and one in a general medical ward, dealing with diabetes, hypertension, those kind of things."

Any change in routine creates a kind of turbulence, and turbulence demands extra time, energy, concentration. At Kwong Wah, as at every health care facility affected by SARS, the meetings and the amount of new information alone added vastly to everyone's burden. Every day at noon, from early March until the end of May, the chief physicians of every department and the head nurses picked up a lunchbox and met at the chief executive's office to hear the latest news coming in from colleagues, from the WHO, the latest word in infection control, the latest treatments being tried. "Everybody was there, so we could make quick decisions. It was a time of great urgency, but it was also a time of friendship. Everyone pulled together."

Tan Tock Seng Hospital in Singapore also held staff briefing sessions twice a day for the first two weeks, circulating updates by email to everyone in the hospital. "We might have had people who would have got frightened and walked out of hospital," said Dr. Brenda Ang. "Fortunately, we didn't have that at all, and everyone just pulled together."

Pulling together happened in several dimensions. In some cases, people in "safe" countries, like Dr. Plant in Australia and Dr. Tom Buckley in New Zealand, signed up to work in SARS-affected countries for the duration. In other cases people who lived in countries with SARS outbreaks but were working in relatively safe areas of medicine volunteered to work in the danger zones. When Tan Tock Seng Hospital put out a call for help as the outbreak began, one of those who responded was Dr. Anuj Gupta, a 28-year-old trainee in internal medicine at the National Neuroscience Institute. For three weeks he worked in the ICU, in full protective gear, alongside three other doctors on the night shift from 5:00 p.m. to 8:00 a.m.

He saw colleagues as young as himself fall sick; he saw an ICU nurse become an ICU patient, and saw the other ICU nurses, who were usually pretty tough, break down in tears. In the three weeks he worked in the ICU he did his best to avoid spreading the virus, keeping to himself, taking his own temperature three times a day, taking vitamins, and getting exercise and rest to boost his immunity. Still, he had two scares—once when his own mother, visiting from India, developed a cough and fever and he had to sit beside her as an ambulance drove her to Tan Tock Seng, and once when he himself developed the same symptoms, but both cases turned out to be false alarms.

What made him decide to volunteer, he told the *Straits Times*, was that his head of department, Dr. T. Umapathi, signed up for a transfer to Tan Tock Seng, despite having two young children. There were also moral issues at play. Doctors, he pointed out, can choose whether to volunteer or not. "But the hospital cleaners and amahs, they don't have that choice."

"It was all crisis and emergency," said Dr. David Hui of the Prince of Wales Hospital in Hong Kong, "but [a decisive factor was that] the senior members of the department all took part in the battle against SARS. My department chairman took part in the 'dirty' team. Initially, some of the junior members were reluctant to join the battle; they proposed a [lottery] to decide who should join the dirty team and who should stay as clean team members. But when the department chairman himself set a good example by walking onto the dirty team, then the other members decided to follow suit. So I think team spirit was very important.

"I don't think we were any more courageous than firemen or policemen. We were just carrying out our duty, and if we saw so many of our colleagues being infected, we would not hesitate to enter the battlefield to help."

* * *

SARS forced hospitals to make institutional changes that were almost unthinkably radical. Some countries responded to the need for isolation (and the fact that smaller hospitals simply weren't equipped to handle large numbers of infectious patients) by converting entire hospitals into SARS-specific institutions, such as the Princess Margaret Hospital in Hong Kong, but there were at least three major problems with putting this theory into practice: it required an extraordinary amount of work that needed to be done at once; it created a high-risk environment by putting all the viruses, so to speak, into one basket; and it was impossible to tell ahead of time how many sick people that hospital would be able to handle.

"On 26th March," explained Dr. Lily Chiu, the hospital's chief executive, "the Department of Health called to ask me whether I could transform the whole of the Princess Margaret Hospital into a SARS hospital. Well, I thought, as part of Hong Kong we have the mission and the responsibility if the government asks it of me, so I said okay.

"Our hospital has a capacity of around 1,200 beds, so I said we could take care of up to a thousand SARS patient—but obviously, at that time we were still learning what SARS was.

"I had around two days to prepare my hospital, to change from an acute general hospital into a hospital that only admitted SARS patients.

"So you can imagine, I had to talk with all my department heads-how they were going to plan surgery, orthopedics, neurosurgery, ob/gyn, pediatrics, how they were going to vacate their existing services into nearby hospitals, and so on. A very important issue would be staff consultation, because the staff would be very concerned. We were suddenly changing the nature of the hospital. So there were many staff forums—in large groups, in small groups.

"The other important thing was that we had to plan for infection control measures, because we heard about all these health care workers coming down, and all these stories which everybody was scared about. So there was really quite a hectic preparation to get ready all the personal protective gear, and to set up infection control measures.

"We had a lot of advice from our colleagues, especially from the Prince of Wales hospital, because they had gone through the whole procedure. The Prince of Wales doctors came over to our hospital to run a forum and share with us their experience—how they set up infection control measures, what were the guidelines, what were the essential things. That was two days of preparation.

"At midnight on the evening of the 28th, we started to close our Accident and Emergency Department to all admissions. The following morning, starting at 9 a.m., we started admitting SARS patients from all over Hong Kong.

"We had very strict criteria: all the patients had to be referred from an Accident and Emergency Department of another hospital and fulfill criteria such as the clinical symptoms of fever, X-ray signs, as well as contact history. We also accepted referrals from the Department of Health Surveillance Medical Centre. These were the two sources that were referred to us.

"But that turned out to be at the peak of the Amoy Gardens outbreak. We admitted nearly 600 SARS patients within that first week. When these patients came in, they were pretty sick because, again, it was a learning curve. In the initial periods, people were not aware what SARS was. They had fever, they thought they would just go to the general practitioner, or stay at home and take [an aspirin] or something like that. So by the time they came in, they were very sick, and they ended up going more or less immediately to the Intensive Care Unit. So with 600 patients flooding in, our ICU started to [overflow]. We started with around fourteen beds in our ICU and we rapidly [needed around sixty]. But we didn't have the capacity, so we were only able to open up three wards, which is around forty-three intensive care patients."

This 48-hour conversion involved far more than moving patients and beds. In the West, modern tertiary care hospitals (i.e., those with specialized services in addition to primary care doctors) have a distinct and inflexible modus operandi. Patients get admitted according to a particular chief complaint, and the nature of the complaint dictates whether they are directed to a general medical service, or a surgical one, or one dealing solely with infectious disease, neurology, obstetrics, pediatrics, psychiatry, and so on. Each such service has not only its own space and personnel but its own unique culture and technology, as well as distinct training held by the team members. Asking, for example, a psychiatry floor team of nurses, doctors, and aides to suddenly function as an infectious disease service borders on the fantastic. Even cross-training in seemingly similar services such as adult medicine and pediatric medicine reveals a great deal of variety and usually a steep learning curve. In the medico-legal environment such as that of the United States, a response like that of the Princess Margaret hospital could likely not have been emulated in any situation short of war.

The master plan in Hong Kong to create a flagship SARS hospital foundered on the reality that there was simply not enough surge capacity in the system: the sheer volume of patients created breakdown. This situation was echoed elsewhere—notably in Toronto, where the Walker Report would insist on the need for surge capacity to be built into the system for the future.

"Prior to that rush of patients we were able to maintain zero infection rate in our health care workers," said Dr. Chiu, "but within that short week, we were unable to make very detailed planning. As you can imagine, we were rushing patients out as well as patients pouring in. We had to gather staff from other hospitals to help out, especially in the Intensive Care Unit. Within that chaotic situation that week, our staff came falling down. And the unfortunate thing was that twenty-five of our ICU staff fell sick because of the initial chaos, the many high-risk procedures and because of the heavy viral load."

Every aspect of hospital life was disrupted. As staff in general wards and respiratory specialties fell sick, staff in other departments would be drafted and have to learn new skills on the job, or would have to give up space, and work extra hours or reschedule patients. Air conditioning was turned off to avoid spreading the virus. Routine cleaning and maintenance took on new significance. Even an aspect of hospital life that would normally have been fairly routine, such as admission, was infinitely more complicated. It took more time, more space, more skill, more equipment, more risk.

"We organized a triage ward on Ward 8D to sort out those cases that were not yet obvious," said Dr. David Hui of the Prince of Wales Hospital. (Similar strategies were used in many other countries: the need to carry out accurate triage under isolated conditions was paramount.) "Someone might develop fever, there might be a patch of pneumonia, but we had to perform blood tests. With SARS we realized later on that they would have a very low lymphocyte count so we had to use the triage ward to have enough time to sort out some of the patients. Some patients might have high fever and pain, but the initial X-rays might appear quite normal-later on we realized, after seeing enough patients, that 20% of SARS patients might initially have a normal-looking X-ray, and it was only during day three that the pneumonia would become obvious. We had to use the triage ward to house these patients temporarily so we could organize blood tests and even CAT scans to detect early pneumonia. And then after we confirmed, we transferred them to the SARS ward, and we opened more and more SARS wards. At the peak time there were five SARS wards." He chuckled in disbelief. "And in each SARS ward we put about 25 or 26 patients.

"I told you we had 156 in the first two weeks, right? But we only had 22 beds. We had to decide where to open the next ward, where to move our pre-existing stock of patients, how to mobilize the nursing staff. And we had more and more health care workers calling in sick, so it was chaotic."

Infection control also requires isolation rooms and negative pressure rooms—that is, rooms whose air pressure is lower than surrounding rooms, so if a door opens potentially contaminated air does not blow out. The very design of emergency rooms, with open spaces, multiple entrances, beds divided only by curtains, and patients and visitors mingling in hallways, makes it impossible to admit potentially infectious patients safely.

Different countries tried different visitor policies. In many hospitals, the visiting rules became progressively stricter—register, give contact information, wear masks—until they were absolute: no visitors for SARS patients. Other hospitals, such as the Prince of Wales, reasoned that to bar visitors altogether placed an intolerable burden on both patients and their families, and by extension raised the likelihood that someone with the disease would be reluctant to come forward, and in postponing hospitalization became more likely to infect others in the community.

Others found inventive middle ground.

"[Isolation is] difficult for our patients," explained Dr. Ling Ma-Lin of Singapore General Hospital, "so we have set up video phones for them where they could still communicate to their loved ones, and our doctors keep a constant kind of a communication with the patients' relatives to update them."

On top of all this, there was the constant danger that health care workers would infect their own families. Some chose to go into quarantine, just in case. Some were lodged in hotels or hostels, and some slept in the hospital.

Everything was inside out. Hospitals were under siege from within; if things continued to get worse, it felt as if they might implode.

Diagnosis

Diagnosis was one of the greatest challenges of the outbreak. Time and again, the symptoms of SARS were deceptive, often masked by other complaints.

Especially in the first week of the illness, the SARS symptoms might be mild, and if someone was suffering from other complaints those might well be far more vivid and noticeable. Mistakes were made everywhere, even by the most vigilant.

"Even if someone didn't meet the case definitions but they looked like they could have [SARS] we would make sure that they were treated as if they had SARS," Barbara Yaffe, acting Medical Officer of Health for the city of Toronto, said. "There were precautions, the contacts were quarantined, the whole caboodle. But there were a number of people that just never hit the radar screen, right? They were totally unrecognized. You probably know we had two phases in our outbreak. Phase two, by the time it came to our radar it had spread quite a bit, because it started probably with a 96-year-old man who had a fractured pelvis, and it looked like he had aspiration pneumonia. Nobody thought of SARS. Nobody thought of anything. And it spread quite a lot before anybody thought of it. Once they think of it-even think of it—they deal with it as if it is SARS."

*SARS Case Definition: from the U.S. Centers for Disease Control**

In the absence of person-to-person transmission of SARS-CoV anywhere in the world, the diagnosis of SARS-CoV disease should be considered only in patients who require hospitalization for radiographically confirmed pneumonia and who have an epidemiologic history that raises the suspicion of SARS-CoV disease. The suspicion for SARS-CoV disease is raised if, within 10 days of symptom onset, the patient:

- Has a history of recent travel to mainland China, Hong Kong, or Taiwan or close contact[1] with ill persons with a history of recent travel to such areas, OR
- Is employed in an occupation at particular risk for SARS-CoV exposure, including a healthcare worker with direct patient contact or a worker in a laboratory that contains live SARS-CoV, OR
- Is part of a cluster of cases of atypical pneumonia without an alternative diagnosis

Once person-to-person transmission of SARS-CoV has been documented in the world, the diagnosis should still be considered in patients who require hospitalization for pneumonia and who have the epidemiologic history described above. In addition, all patients with fever or lower respiratory symptoms (e.g., cough, shortness of breath, difficulty breathing) should be questioned about whether within 10 days of symptom onset they have had:

- Close contact with someone suspected of having SARS-CoV disease, OR
- A history of foreign travel (or close contact with an ill person with a history of travel) to a location with documented or suspected SARS-CoV, OR
- Exposure to a domestic location with documented or suspected SARS-CoV (including a laboratory that contains live SARS-CoV), or close contact with an ill person with such an exposure history.

[1]Close contact: A person who has cared for or lived with a person with SARS-CoV disease or had a high likelihood of direct contact with respiratory secretions and/or body fluids of a person with SARS-CoV disease. Examples of close contact include kissing or hugging, sharing eating or drinking utensils, talking within 3 feet, and direct touching. Close contact does not include activities such as walking by a person or briefly sitting across a waiting room or office.

**Accessed July 2004. Please check CDC SARS website for the most up-to-date information. The above is not intended as a substitute for a physician's opinion nor should it be used as medical advice.*

The hyper-vigilance in itself became a problem. In Singapore, a case of dengue fever was missed because doctors were looking for SARS.

"We had a lot of that," said Dr. Bonnie Henry, one of Toronto's Associate Medical Officers of Health. "People were testing everybody for SARS and forgetting to test for tuberculosis and all the other things that cause illness. We had 24 cases of TB identified in the first month of the outbreak after we reminded physicians to look for other more common illnesses."

Looking for SARS, however, was harder than looking for most diseases.

"There was no blood test to diagnose SARS until April," said David Hui of the Prince of Wales hospital. "It was only on the first of April that we started to have PCR (polymerase chain reaction, a gene-amplification methodology) available on the naso-pharyngeal aspirate, and the serology (blood test) was only available at the end of April. So for the first month we were fighting in the dark, relying on clinical observations. I had to observe my patients from the bedside three to four times a day."

Even the PCR and blood tests, though, were slow and not entirely reliable. By the time the outbreak ended, there was still no quick, reliable lab test that could be used to diagnose SARS—in fact, even after the outbreak was over, during an event in British Columbia where several elderly residents of a nursing home developed respiratory illness, the lab tests came back positive when the patients clearly did not have SARS.

(In laboratory medicine, the concepts of sensitivity and specificity become especially important. In a population of 100 people, of whom 20 carry disease X, a sensitive test is one which can detect all 20, leaving no positive person undiagnosed. The price for all this sensitivity is usually an overdiagnosis: it may actually register 25 people as having the condition—i.e., 5 extra, or 5 false-positives. That's where specificity comes in. A specific test will not register any false positives. However, it may well give false negatives. In the above example, a specific test for condition X may actually give a result of 15: under-representing the truth by 5, or 5 false-negatives. The SARS tests turned out to initially have greater sensitivity than specificity-useful for a screening test, where one can afford to treat a few uninfected people, rather than let truly infected people escape the net.)

As a result, all over the world health care workers had to rely on what might be called "diagnosis by epidemiology." If you had flu or pneumonia symptoms and you had come into contact with someone with SARS, you automatically became SARS-likely.

Unfortunately, this caused two important problems. First, it created a vast, almost infinite amount of work tracking the movements and contacts of everyone who had or probably had SARS. Second, it meant that no lab test could quickly give anyone a clean bill of health, so anyone who lived near a SARS case, or had come from a SARS region, was under a cloud of mistrust that could not readily be dispelled.

The whole process of diagnosis never ceased to be, to some degree, a makeshift one, and potentially misleading.

Dr. Bonnie Henry of Toronto, Dr. Donald Low, Professor of Medicine and Microbiology at the University of Toronto, and Dr. Tony Mazzulli, a microbiologist from Mount Sinai (NY), went to North York Hospital to assess a couple of psychiatric patients who looked like SARS cases but for whom no epidemiological link could be found. Mazzulli and Henry thought the patients had SARS, while Low did not. As was common practice, the patients were isolated just in case.

A few days later, a lab test found Mycoplasma, a pathogen that is a common cause of pneumonia, suggesting that the SARS virus was not the cause of the psychiatric patients' illness.

After several weeks passed, though, blood tests showed that one patient had developed antibodies to the SARS coronavirus (SARS-CoV), which strongly suggested he had been a SARS case—but while a stool sample from the same patient tested positive for the SARS coronavirus, the PCR test was negative.

"Somebody help me!" Low said later. "Could somebody please make something straightforward here?"

No epidemiological link was ever established to connect the psychiatric patients with any known SARS contact.

Treatment

In the beginning, everyone was in the dark, trying one course of treatment, then trying another, watching the caseload mounting daily.

"We gave our colleagues Tamiflu [an anti-influenza medication] on the assumption that it was some sort of unusual influenza," said Dr.

David Hui of the Prince of Wales Hospital, "but they did not respond. We also added very broad-spectrum antibiotics [to cover bacterial rather than viral agents]. Again, none of them improved."

Doctors could only keep trying treatments, watch the virus play its hand, and compare notes.

"It took us about three weeks to learn from the first batch of patients," David Hui explained. "Gradually, we recognized the clinical course of the disease."

The disease turned out to have several distinct phases. The first involved high fever, pain, a general feeling of not being well, and one small patch of pneumonia. At the beginning of the second week, the pneumonia suddenly began to spread to both lungs, and the patient developed severe respiratory failure. One patient in two would need supplemental oxygen. One patient in four would have such trouble breathing that he or she would need to be sent to the I.C.U. One in eight had such difficulty breathing that he or she could no longer manage alone, and needed artificial help from a mechanical ventilator, forcing oxygen down a tube inserted into the lungs, a process called intubation.

"Every day there were two to three meetings among the clinicians, consisting of myself, infectious disease fellows, gastro-enterologists, microbiologists and radiologists, and we sat down and went through every case in detail—blood counts, X-rays. After the first few days when the patients failed to respond to Tamiflu, we realized that it had to be something viral, so the microbiologists recommended Ribavirin [another anti-viral medication used for influenza]. At the time it was the only anti-viral with some track record against DNA and RNA viruses. Everyone, including Toronto, was using Ribavirin. It was only weeks later that we were told that there was no in vitro activity." In other words, Ribavirin didn't help.

"In the second week we took some CAT scans and found some ground-glass changes that mimicked a condition called BOOP (bronchiolitis obliterans organizing pneumonia). We'd seen that condition many times before in rheumatology patients—for example, patients who have lupus—and that (BOOP) usually was responsive to steroids. So during the second week, when we had so many patients deteriorating, developing pneumonia on both lungs and developing ground-glass on the computer scan, we started to use steroids, and to our surprise it worked."

Many patients who'd needed oxygen began to breathe better, and the white shadows on their X-rays shrank.

Note: These are cortisone steroids, not the anabolic steroids used (illegally) by athletes to gain muscle mass. Used over short periods in small to moderate doses, they promote tissue healing and can suppress inflammatory reactions. Used over a long period in large doses, though, they can cause bone damage and actually weaken the immune system, among other unpleasant side-effects.

When the initial group of health care workers began to improve, "we asked them to donate their serum, which contained neutralizing antibodies to the SARS virus."

Serum is the contents of the blood, minus the red cells, which were returned to the donor patient.

"We transfused the serum from the recovering patients to those who were still deteriorating and to our surprise it actually helped." Patients no longer needed steroids, or needed only reduced dosages.

In a sense Hui and his colleagues were lucky to be in the same hospital as the recovering patients, so they could have easy access to their serum, and as a result they used much lower levels of steroids than any other hospital. This would turn out to be a significant issue, because especially in China some recovered patients who had been treated with very high doses of steroids over prolonged periods turned out to have vascular necrosis of the long bones—an estimated 30% of cases in Beijing, 13% overall in Hong Kong. At the Prince of Wales Hospital, he said, they have conducted 220 MRI bone scans and found only 8 patients with vascular necrosis—probably because of the availability of the convalescent plasma. Even by the end of the outbreak, though, there were recommended courses of treatment but no guarantees and no cures. All the same, SARS was a more familiar enemy. Epidemiologists were beginning to understand and explain how it spread, which helped enormously in the process of containment. Children were turning out to be curiously resistant to the virus, which led some researchers to wonder whether some of the damage to the lungs was caused by the adults' own immune response, which in children was not yet fully developed. It was becoming clearer at what times patients were most infectious, and how the virus might be passed on. But there was no silver bullet: what mattered was keeping the patients alive until their own immune systems could cope, and keeping the virus from spreading.

Infection Control

"From the tenth of March we were already wearing surgical masks and gloves," said David Hui, "but on the eleventh of March we were starting to use N95 masks [a particular type of infection control mask used in dealing with TB among other respiratory conditions] because we realized that there was something unusual. In fact, when I look back, we had the index case who came in on the 4th of March who went to visit a friend in the Metropole on the 21st of February. Two days later [February 23], he started to feel sick, but he wasn't admitted to our hospital until the 4th of March. When he came in he only had right upper lobe pneumonia. He was under the care of my friend who is a hematologist on duty for general medicine, but he had persistent fever despite broad-spectrum antibiotics [which would help reverse a bacterial pneumonia]. I was consulted on the tenth of March to see this index case, and I was actually invited to perform a bronchoscopy on this guy [which entails putting a small tube into the lungs and taking a washing or sample of the area for diagnostic purposes]. I walked in with a surgical mask and gloves, and I looked at the X-rays. Fortunately, his fever was starting to settle, and the X-ray was starting to improve, so I decided not to perform the bronchoscopy.

"In retrospect, I was very lucky, because in February 2003 my friend in Guangzhou and his team performed a bronchoscopy on a patient with SARS and fourteen health care workers got infected."

Infection control was at the heart of SARS. Without a vaccine or a treatment, it was what the outbreak was all about: effective infection control would contain SARS; ineffective infection control would not only spread it, but by spreading it among health care workers would be the worm in the core of a nation's medical defenses.

* * *

One of the many insidious features of SARS was the fact that the very technologies that were needed to save the lives of patients turned out to endanger the lives of the doctors and nurses around them, and in fact anyone in the hospital.

The explosion of cases at the beginning of the Prince of Wales outbreak seems to have been caused, or at least facilitated by a standard piece of general medical equipment, familiar to any parent whose infant has severe asthma: a nebulizer.

"The index case, the 26-year-old, was admitted on the fourth of March," explained Hui. "My friend gave him nebulized Ventolin [albuterol, a common anti-asthma drug] from the 6th of March to the 12th."

A nebulizer is a pump that forces liquid medication through a nozzle, converting it into a mist. The mist is in turn forced down a tube into a mask that the patient wears, so he or she breathes in a mixture of air and medication. Albuterol acts on the airways, helping them relax and widen, and also freeing up the cilia, hair-like projections lining the airway, which can help mucus to be coughed up more easily.

But the nebulizer is not a closed system: the mask needs exhaust holes, or the whole device, driven by the pump, would inflate like a balloon. These holes or vents are quite sizeable—Hui reckons that a good 80% of the medication is actually wasted by escaping through the vents—and once the patient would start to cough, exhaled air from his or her lungs would escape into the ward.

Ironically, one of the difficulties with identifying SARS and getting sputum samples for diagnosis was that the disease produces a dry rather than a phlegm-filled cough and the virus is oddly reclusive, establishing itself deep in one of the lobes. The nebulized Ventolin had the doubly unfortunate effect of (a) flushing it out of its hiding place and (b) converting its vehicle from a truck into a sports car. Coughed or sneezed out in droplet form, the virus had an effective radius of only a few feet. Converted into an aerosol mist, it could travel much farther. Three of the early SARS patients in the Prince of Wales Hospital were cardiologists who actually had nothing to do with the index patient, and had merely visited the ward.

The layout and design of the ward itself added to the problems with infection control, creating a kind of captive audience for the spread of the virus.

"In those days, we had a [large] general ward. You know, you put 36 patients in one ward without any partitions, just curtains to separate the patients; the beds would be less than a meter apart, and the airflow [through the air conditioning] would only be about three air exchanges per hour.

"But we had no idea about this before SARS. Nobody knew. And the index case was only identified on the 13th of March when his mother, brother, sister, and domestic helper developed flu-like illness.

We realized the index case had to be him, so he was isolated straight away in the only single room of Ward 8A on the 13th of March."

Hospitals could stop using nebulizers, but they couldn't stop using another technology that turned out to help spread the virus: intubation. This usually is a life-saving procedure for which the patient is sedated and paralyzed. In this case, wrestling the tube down the patient's throat, with the patient coughing and sometimes struggling, seems to have forced virus-laden moisture out of the recesses of the patient's lungs, broadcasting out among the half-dozen health care workers clustering around and bending over the bed.

The greatest danger arose when patients in open wards deteriorated so rapidly that they needed to be intubated there and then: an emergency intubation is such a hasty and invasive operation that the patient often coughs hard and often, and to do so in a general ward was potentially disastrous. Toronto got suspicious when six of eight people in the room during an intubation got sick, including the anaesthesiologist [who sometimes performs the actual procedure]. Some hospitals dealt with the problem by sedating the patients before intubating them. The Prince of Wales Hospital responded by trying to avoid the haste.

"We tried very hard not to use emergency intubation because the health care workers would be at high risk if we had to intubate urgently.

"Because it was such a highly infectious disease, with so many health care workers in our institution being infected, what we decided at the very beginning was that if we gave them five liters of oxygen by nasal cannula, and if we still were unable to maintain their oxygen saturation of 90% [greater than 90% is good], and the patient started to have a very fast respiratory rate, then we would send them to intensive care to avoid emergency intubation. In other words, we transferred them to ICU electively. Very fortunately, at the Prince of Wales we had no emergency intubations.

"We were very lucky. In other hospitals such catastrophes did occur. I heard that there was one hospital where one patient was intubated as an emergency but there was no bed in the ICU. One doctor and one male nurse had to [support] the patient for several hours, and both got SARS and both eventually died."

* * *

Meanwhile, even the routine and (dangerously) unconsidered acts of hygiene had to be rigorously enforced—and here SARS served as a wake-up call for the health care systems of the world, because hospital hygiene had become an area of medicine that had long been taken for granted, and had fallen into a state of mental and institutional disrepair.

Infections are often said to be opportunistic, and SARS was opportunistic in a slightly different way, breeding in overlooked and unconsidered areas of public health. As the Walker Report (For the Public's Health: The Initial Report of the Ontario Expert Panel on SARS and Infectious Disease Control, produced by the Ontario Ministry of Health and Long-Term Care) summed the situation up, "infection control is invisible until an outbreak occurs."

The Walker Report treated infection control as one of its highest priorities, mincing no words: "[I]n many cases, health care facilities faced with a range of competing demands have placed less importance on infectious disease control and have demonstrated limited compliance with even basic prevention and control techniques, such as handwashing." It criticized "sub-optimal level of infection control training, staffing and accountability," and blamed not only a lack of funding for infection control but a lack of training, even a lack of trained people who could conduct training, and courses for those who would like to become infection control practitioners. In 1985, the Expert Panel noted, the CDC in Atlanta recommended that there be a minimum of one infection control practitioner for every 250 acute care beds. In 2001, the Canadian Infection Prevention and Control Alliance raised the bar to one practitioner per 150-175 acute care beds. In 2002, a third professional body recommended a ratio of 1:100 or 1:120. It further advised that "recent research has shown that the vast majority of acute care facilities do not meet the 2001 standard and almost half do not even meet the now-obsolete 1985 standard."

One health care worker interviewed by the Expert Panel said, "SARS certainly illustrated the need for increased awareness of infectious diseases, and showed us all how quickly an entire health care system could be shut down. It showed us how unprepared we are in our ability to contain and control not only new and emerging diseases, but those such as influenza and tuberculosis."

As the report points out, SARS was a dramatic illustration of a problem that has been steadily growing, but lacked attention. In other words, it was all just another systems problem to eventually be addressed—but then people started dying.

"SARS is the tip of the iceberg of the largely unrecognized problem of facility-acquired infections... In developed countries, about 5-10% of patients in acute care hospitals acquire an infection that was not present on admission. In the United States, hospital-acquired infections are the second most frequent type of adverse incident occurring in hospitals—second only to medication errors.

"The precise rate of facility-acquired infection in Canada is not known [but]... it is estimated that there are 220,000 occurrences of facility-acquired infections in Canadian hospitals annually, resulting in excess of 8,000 deaths. "The number of occurrences appears to be on the increase, partly due to a surge in the number of antibiotic-resistant pathogens. For example, 440 identified cases of methicillin-resistant Staphylococcus aureus (MRSA) were found in 20 of the 21 Canadian hospitals and long-term care facilities studied... in 1995 over an 18-month period. More recent studies have shown that the rate of MRSA infections has increased 10-fold over the past decade."

The CDC has estimated the annual cost of hospital-acquired infections in the US to be $5 billion.

In *The New Killer Diseases*, Elinor Levy and Mark Fischetti write: "Infection and drug resistance are rampant in hospitals because of the unique ecosystem inside their walls. There is a concentration of infectious patients, a large number of highly susceptible patients whose immune systems are already stressed from other illnesses or surgery, and numerous operating tables, patient beds, nurses' counters, and instruments that are constantly bombarded with germs. Drugs are administered heavily [thereby promoting the development of drug-resistant pathogens]. And doctors and nurses too often touch infectious organisms on one person and carry them to the next. The higher the density of these factors, the greater the risk; patients in intensive-care units are five to ten times more likely than other hospital patients to pick up an infection."

Levy and Fischetti cite a study conducted in Switzerland by researchers in the Infection Control Program at the University of Geneva Hospitals. By persuading doctors and nurses to increase their rate of handwashing merely from 48% to 66 % of the times they should do so, they reduced the rate of in-house infection from 16.9% to 9.9%, and the transmission of MRSA dropped by more than 50%.

* * *

During the SARS outbreak, sloppy hospital hygiene was potentially fatal.

"What has changed tremendously," said Dr. Ling of Singapore General, "is the heightened awareness and the daily mandatory temperature checks—in fact for us it's three times a day for our staff. [That], and having to put on the various protective apparel, gown, gloves, masks and everything—that's something very new for all of us." In Tan Tock Seng, infection control nurses worked overtime making sure that masks fitted properly, from nurses through people who came to fix the air conditioning, "down to mortuary attendants because again we were not sure whether there was still likely to be a viral spread even after the patient was dead," recalled Dr. Brenda Ang. "In a way it was not difficult to get compliance because this was an unknown, it was frightening. In fact, a lot of people wanted to do more than what we were recommending. Compliance was not an issue at all."

Garry Smyth, a videographer who visited the theater of the SARS war for the WHO, and a veteran of an Ebola outbreak, gave a vivid outsider's perspective of the demands made by full barrier nursing.

"In Beijing I wore three layers of clothing, which included a one-piece jump suit that made movement so limited I could not bend down and put on my foot coverings." He was so hot he couldn't breathe. Eventually he and the hospital staff compromised: he was allowed to wear only two masks, a N95 and a surgical mask. The nurse, meanwhile, was wearing three pairs of gloves. "People were wearing that for six hour shifts."

He showed me a photo shot in the ICU of two people, him and the nurse, in drab-aqua gowns, hoods, full body suit, goggles. Even the videocamera is swaddled in a sleeve which he cut off a gown, with the elastic cuff around the lens. When he finished he threw the sleeve away and disinfected the lens and the viewfinder, the only exposed parts.

One of the hardest things for staff working under full protective gear, he said, was to avoid touching one's eyes. "I was wearing goggles, and they kept fogging up. I had to keep shaking my head to get drops to form so I could see." Even taking off the apron and gown without touching their external surfaces, and taking off one glove so that it ends up inside out, inside the other glove, is a tricky business.

Ideal equipment was often not available. United Christian Hospital (UCH) was one of the worst-hit hospitals in Hong Kong, with 26 medical workers infected in the wake of the outbreak at nearby Amoy Gardens. At UCH, one doctor wore the same mask for so long he wore a hole in it. Medical workers were supposed to change their N95 masks after every shift, but supplies were so tight the staff took to wearing them for seven days, unless they were wet or contaminated. Surgical caps ran out, so they were issued regular shower caps; protective gowns were in such short supply the staff resorted to wearing regular surgical gowns, even though they offered less protection.

Part of the SARS legacy, then, was a wake-up call: nobody expected that hospital infection control was so porous, nor that its failings could be so dangerous. An entire overlooked dimension of health care had been revealed.

In the Geneva headquarters of the WHO, Garry Smyth shared a film he made of an amazing demonstration of the importance of infection control. He had two doctors working on intubating a dummy, which had a small amount of gel smeared around the lips and chin to simulate "respiratory secretions." The gel was formulated to be more or less invisible under normal conditions, but show up under ultra-violet light.

The whole sequence was filmed live, and Smyth didn't know how effective a demonstration it would be. In the back of his mind he half-expected they'd need to set up a staged version to make the point more effectively.

The physicians finished the intubation, which took about five minutes, then Smyth turned off the lights.

"It was unreal. It was only then that it clicked how many times the doctor and nurse had touched that dummy's head and chin. We looked and said, 'What the hell is that?'"

What they saw appears on the screen: eerie patches of light blue are glowing everywhere—on the protective clothing; on the surgical tools used and set aside on a tray; on a couple of syringes with the rims, plungers and barrels all glowing. "It was just incredible."

He froze the shot on the cardiac monitor, where the switches were glowing. Even if the doctor disrobed and disinfected after finishing the procedure, someone else—even the cleaning staff—was going to end up touching that heart monitor. And the SARS coronavirus can survive outside the body for up to two days.

* * *

Dr. Andrew Yip, sitting in his office in Kwong Wah Hospital in shirt and tie with his mask slung under his chin, reflected on the events of a year ago.

He says that when he heard the Department of Health alerts about atypical pneumonia in Guangdong, his attitude was, "If it comes, Hong Kong can probably handle it. Obviously," he went on, shaking his head and laughing grimly, "I was wrong. It totally changed my outlook as a clinician. SARS ripped through any health care system. Look at Canada. None of us expected anything so infectious, so contagious. SARS caught us all by surprise."

He shook his head, as if still shell-shocked.

Chapter 10.

The Worst Days: A Near Miss

What was it like to have SARS?

On March 14, Ken Ching, a banker from Singapore, met with four of his colleagues to decide whether they should visit their bank's branches in China and Hong Kong.

It was a pivotal time. Just the day before, the Singapore government had advised against unnecessary travel to both places. On the other hand, only some fifty cases of this new "atypical pneumonia" had been reported in Hong Kong, so, they thought, perhaps the situation wasn't that serious.

"There was no cause for alarm at that time," Ching later told the *Straits Times*. "There was only a travel advisory. [There was] a job to be done and someone had to do it."

The group was split: two decided it was too dangerous to go, but Ching and two colleagues, a man and a woman (the team leader), decided to go to Hong Kong. Just in case, they decided to get a flu vaccination—which might not do any good against SARS, they realized, but might boost the immune system or their morale. Just in case, they took a thermometer, face masks, and flu pills.

When they landed in Hong Kong, nothing looked out of the ordinary apart from a group of Taiwanese tourists wearing masks.

"I had expected a lot of checks, but it was business as usual. The taxi drivers wore no masks. We took a bus—no one wore masks."

They stayed at the Park Lane Hotel, in the ultra-high-rise district at the heart of downtown Hong Kong; the Fifth Avenue or Park Lane of the city. Hong Kong itself also seemed just the same as always: crowded and bustling. The whole SARS thing must just be the usual media exaggeration, they figured. They went out for dinner, and just to be sure, all three took anti-flu tablets before going to bed.

The following morning the team leader rang him after breakfast to tell him that her temperature was a little high—37.6 degrees (99.7

Fahrenheit). Ching told her it might just be because of the coffee she just had. They went to work at the bank's branch office and settled into a pattern that lasted for the rest of the week: work, dinner, then back to the hotel.

During the team's second week in Hong Kong, the city was transformed. The SARS count rose from 50 to 367; schools shut down; more than 1,600 people were ordered into quarantine. In the bank, the trio from Singapore found that their Hong Kong colleagues were starting to keep them at arm's length for a reason that two weeks previously would have made no sense: they were staying in a hotel.

SARS created a temporary and very specific form of xenophobia. Word had already got out that the virus had first been passed to a Hong Kong citizen—and to people from a range of other countries—in a hotel. For the next few months, hotels took on a new identity as what might be called a nexus of transmission, a virus junction.

Still, work went on in the Hong Kong bank office, though the office manager ordered the cleaners to visit more often, planned for disaster contingencies, and ordered anyone who was sick or coughing to go to the doctor. A box of sixty face masks was ordered (at a price that had already tripled) and handed out to the staff. Both of Ching's Singapore colleagues took to wearing masks to and from work, but he refused, thinking they were unnecessary. The three of them decided not to eat dinner out anymore, however.

"Out of 15 people crossing the road, we counted more than half of them wearing masks. We started ordering takeaway and stopped e ating in public areas," Ching said. "I started walking very fast in crowded places. No nightspots, no parties, no restaurants. Anyone coughed, we left a place. Anyone sneezed, we left."

On Wednesday everyone was passing the word: SARS had broken out in Amoy Gardens. The first three things that sprang to mind when Ching heard the news were: Is Amoy Gardens near the Park Lane Hotel? Is it near our office? Do we have to go past it?

It's a curious (and perhaps significant) geographical and demographic fact that SARS sprang up across the narrow strait in Kowloon and the New Territories, which are more residential, poorer, and closer to mainland China, and rarely jumped the half-mile or so to Hong Kong Island, the business and shopping heart of Hong Kong. Amoy Gardens was nowhere near Ching's office or the hotel, but the situation was getting very tense. The team discussed cutting the visit short, but decided to stay as they had only three more days to go.

By the time they did leave, on Saturday, March 29, Hong Kong airport was a combat zone.

"Everyone was wearing a mask, even the security guards, the counter girl, and the Customs officers."

The team leader, who had worn her mask religiously for most of the week, was looking ill. She had been coughing on and off for several days, and complaining of a sore throat. At check-in, she told the others she'd better not sit with them, and moved to an aisle seat at the back of the plane, where she slept with her mask on.

On his first day back in Singapore, a Sunday, Ching started coughing. The following day he started feeling as if he had the flu, and his temperature went up. On Tuesday evening he went to see a doctor. When he told the staff that he had just got back from Hong Kong, they left the room so they could put their masks on.

"My temperature was 38 degrees C. The doctor wrote a letter and told me to go to Tan Tock Seng," the designated SARS hospital. "I couldn't believe it."

What he called "the worst days" of his life were beginning. He was at Tan Tock Seng within the hour, where he was met by nurses in gowns, gloves, and masks. They gave him a mask, took his temperature, drew blood, and X-rayed his chest.

Nothing seemed to be wrong. The staff at Tan Tock Seng sent him home with medication and told him to stay there under home quarantine.

Over the next few days, his temperature was up and down. On Thursday the critical public health intervention took place: he was called by a nurse from Tan Tock Seng—five times.

On the first call, the nurse asked his temperature. Ching admitted that it was high.

On the second call, the nurse asked at which hotel Ching and his colleagues had stayed in Hong Kong. The Park Lane, he said. She in turn told him that an Indonesian boy living in Singapore had caught SARS at the Park Lane. Contact tracing had caught up with him.

Shortly afterwards, the nurse called back. On which floor had they stayed? "Eighth and ninth," Ching replied. "Which floor was the boy staying on?"

The nurse didn't answer.

The fourth call was more peremptory. "We are sending an ambulance to pick you up," the nurse said. Ching said he would drive himself.

The nurse called back. "Okay, drive yourself. But come now, or we'll come and get you."

As soon as he got to Tan Tock Seng, the staff took another X-ray of his chest. He sat in a corner while three doctors pored over it. Ching kept thinking about what to have for dinner, thinking that he wouldn't be one of "the cases," thinking he'd be home soon. Nurses gave him bread and mineral water. After he had been there for more than two hours, a doctor detached himself from the huddle around his X-ray and came over to say, "We have to isolate you."

"I told him: 'No, I am not staying in [the] hospital.' They had the wrong guy, I was not sick and I would be a good boy, I would confine myself at home."

No dice. A nurse led him to an ambulance, which ferried him the short distance from Tan Tock Seng to the Communicable Disease Centre.

* * *

The Communicable Disease Centre looked more like a prison than a hospital.

"My room had an attached toilet, a manual-dial television set and pillows wrapped in plastic. A row of windows had been thrown open and the ceiling fan was spinning at full blast. There were two disposal bins, one for regular garbage and the other for contaminated gowns and such. The nurse told me I could press the bell if I wanted anything and I was not to turn off the fan."

The thought that he was trapped with other SARS patients scared him. He refused to change into a Communicable Disease Centre T-shirt, insisted on wearing his own shirt, nearly broke the TV, demanded they go out and buy him fish ball noodles for supper.

"One of the nurses raided a few lockers of her colleagues and found chicken-flavored cup noodles for me. I was very moved, so I ate it," he said.

He tried to sleep, but medical staff came in twice during the night to draw blood. The patient next door coughed constantly.

"I heard someone cry, I don't know where from. That night was the worst. I was miserable. I was lonely."

At nine the next morning, he was seen by three doctors, who had some provisionally good news: his temperature was down to 37 degrees (98.6 Fahrenheit), and if it stayed there, he could be discharged by Saturday.

His girlfriend brought him clothes, magazines, and that essential twenty-first century accessory: his cell phone charger. His uncle brought him yong tau foo (a spicy fish-paste dish) and sugar cane juice. Neither, though, was allowed to see him: everything had to be handed over via the nursing staff.

"I thought about getting out of there, of what I would do if tested positive for SARS. I thought if I died in there, the last my parents would see of me would be my ashes.

"The doctor was frank. He said I had to fight the illness myself. The pills could only suppress the fever. He told me that a young man like me would walk out of that place. That pushed me on through the next two nights."

On Saturday morning, he was still hoping to be discharged until a nurse asked him what he would like to eat for lunch—and dinner.

"My tears almost flowed out again. I told them I wasn't going to have lunch or dinner. I was checking out today."

For whatever reason, the Communicable Disease Centre staff changed their minds: he was told he could leave after lunch. He called his girlfriend and uncle and shaved for the first time since he had entered the building.

"A nurse walked past and asked: 'Mr. Ching, why are you shaving?' I said I was going home. They all came over, combed my hair, poured me water, packed my things. Then, they arranged for an ambulance to take me back to Tan Tock Seng to pick up my car.

"I came out and thanked all the nurses. My nurse came up to me and said: 'Don't come back. We are very tired.' They had tears in their eyes. Even the security guard told me to take care of myself."

* * *

Ken Ching never found out for certain whether or not he had had full-blown SARS. Over the next week, he was mostly struck by how lightly he had taken the threat of the virus, how vain he had been in refusing to wear a mask.

Ten days after he had left the Communicable Disease Centre, Ken Ching went back, and the staff drew three vials of blood. He waited four hours. Finally a doctor came over.

He was in the clear.

Chapter 11.

Racing the Virus

Ever since James Watson wrote *The Double Helix*, the public has been treated to a series of books about scientific races, some involving the most brilliant minds at work, the most intractable problems, and calling even the very meaning of life in question. In all these profound and meaningful endeavors, there was and is the ever-present backdrop of the papers to be published, the careers to be launched, the Nobel prizes to be won—all trappings of the very real competition in science.

SARS took that formula and rewrote it backwards, even inside out. There was certainly competition, but at least for a while there was an unusual and possibly unique element of global cooperation, a potentially fragile coalition held together by one man who didn't even have his own lab. At least for a while it seemed as if the future of humankind might be at stake, but in the end the discovery of the culprit virus and the sequencing of its genome hasn't (yet) provided a cure, or a vaccine, or even a cheap and effective diagnostic test.

Even the medals table was strangely inverted: the lab that is now widely acknowledged as first having identified the SARS coronavirus actually reached the finish line fifth, and even then there was a photo finish and the equivalent of a steward's inquiry. Two labs that beat it to the post got the wrong answer. The first lab to publicly identify the pathogen also got the wrong answer; and in doing so it buried the work of an entirely different lab that had got the right answer before anyone, but its researchers never published their results for fear of being punished.

The story begins, not surprisingly, in China, and it begins with what will become a familiar complaint: the inability to get hold of specimens for testing. The Chinese Center for Disease Control and Prevention in Beijing (another organization abbreviated to CDC, like its U.S. namesake) had difficulty getting doctors in Guangdong province to send them samples. Throughout the outbreak, there would be complaints about favoritism and insider trading of specimens of lung tissue or respiratory secretions: not only was there competition to help humankind, there was also prestige at stake; to add to the difficulties, it proved to be a difficult virus to obtain. Some viruses multiply in the blood and are found easily enough. Some respiratory viruses teem in the mucus and respiratory secretions. The SARS coronavirus (SARS CoV) typically lurked in one lobe, deep in a lung, and the symptoms it provoked involved a dry cough that produced no mucus,nNot to mention that getting close to a sick patient could be quite hazardous to the researcher's health.

Eventually a few specimens arrived. First plague and Legionnaire's disease were ruled out and then, on February 18, 2003, Dr. Hong Tao, a senior microbiologist at CDC's Institute for Virology and a member of the Chinese Academy of Engineering, announced that the culprit was chlamydia. One strain of the chlamydia bacterium causes a well-known sexually transmitted disease, but two others can cause respiratory infection.

In point of fact, chlamydia was never a convincing candidate, for a number of reasons. Physicians who had actually treated SARS patients, such as the respected Dr. Zhong Nanshan, the director of the Institute for Respiratory Diseases in Guangzhou, knew that it didn't respond to antibiotics, so it was unlikely to be bacterial. The sample size (seven patients) was very small, given the difficulty of getting specimens. In addition, Hong couldn't actually isolate the pathogen or get antibodies to chlamydia to react to the tissue samples. In two of those tissue samples, however, Hong found a coronavirus—later to be unmasked as the true villain. The only convincing elements of the announcement were Hong's seniority, his prestige, and the reputation of the institution. In China, these qualities counted for a great deal—so much so that the CDC and the Ministry of Health effectively silenced any other opinions.

"They closed the doors and only thought about chlamydia," said Dr. Henk Bekedam, head of WHO's Beijing office, which was unfortunate and possibly tragic, because at the same time, a team from the Academy of Military Medical Sciences' (AMMS) Institute of Microbiology and Epidemiology, led by Zhu Qingyu and Qin Ede, had just come back from Guangdong with patient samples from military hospitals. By February 22, 2003 (the day Professor Liu was admitted to Kwong Wah Hospital), they had managed to grow a virus from the samples, and four days later, using an electron microscope, they found what looked like particles of a coronavirus. After a few more days of work they discovered that serum from recovering patients, which contained antibodies to the outbreak virus, slowed the growth of the isolated virus, a strong indication that the two were the same. Yet they were bedeviled by the shortage of specimens, and Hong's prestige.

"We wanted to be very sure," one of the AMMS researchers told *Science*. "Dr. Hong Tao is very famous in China. We had to show respect."

It was more than an issue of respect, though: the chlamydia hypothesis had acquired the status of gospel. As late as April 11, when another Chinese CDC researcher confirmed the coronavirus, his department rebuked him and, according to Science, "set up a working group the next day to control publicity about SARS pathogen studies."

Meanwhile, a separate group that could have sequenced the virus was also denied specimens until mid-April—a day after a Canadian group had already sequenced the virus and posted the results online.

* * *

None of this was known to the outside world, though, where a separate set of efforts were under way to find out what was causing this mysterious epidemic.

When the first rumors leaked out of southern China, Hong Kong took the situation seriously enough to begin investigations of its own, led by Professor Kwok-Yung Yuen.

In explaining the chain of events, Yuen, astonishingly young for someone in such a position, mocked himself for being an academic and being unable to talk without writing on the board. Sure enough, everything he said came with a diagram, a keyword, a subdivision into categories.

"What was most alarming to me was that there were doctors and nurses and health care workers coming down with the disease. This is extremely unusual, because they are young, they are immunocompetent," he said, emphasizing "young" and "immunocompetent" on the whiteboard. "You never see doctors and nurses dying of influenza and pneumonia.

"So in the middle of February I called a meeting with my guys in the department on the second floor of the university pathology building. It included Dr. Guan Yi, Dr. Zheng Bo-Jian, and our chief of virology, Professor Malik Peiris. Given the fact that it was flu season, they thought the most likely candidate was a genetically drifted or shifted influenza virus, possibly a variant of the H5N1."

Drs. Guan Yi and Zheng Bo-Jian, potentially risking their lives, went to Guangzhou to see if they could acquire a specimen from any of the pneumonia victims. In Guangzhou they met Zhong Nanshan and his colleagues. "They allowed us to bring specimens back to Hong Kong to look for the agents. At that time everybody was thinking bird flu..."

This turned out to be a trap. The way a virologist looks for a virus is by taking a sample from the infected person—in the case of a pneumonia-like disease, some respiratory secretions—and adds tiny amount of the sample to a growth medium. In the case of bacteria, in can even be the classic Petri dish, but viruses are different from bacteria in this crucial respect: they can only grow and reproduce inside host cells. So the researcher has to provide a single, orderly layer of cells, called a cell line, for the virus to penetrate and inhabit. But viruses are genetically programmed to look for the very specific type of cell that suits them best. An oral herpes virus, for example, breeds only in certain types of skin or nerve cell. Yuen and his lab, suspecting influenza, introduced the Guangzhou samples to a cell line well known to act as a host for influenza viruses. Nothing happened.

Shortly afterwards, and quite unexpectedly, Yuen and his team were presented with another sample, this time from a lot closer to home: from the Kwong Wah Hospital in Kowloon, provided by the unfortunate Professor Liu. Again they tried to grow up an influenza virus; again nothing happened.

In a sense, this was useful information, because now they could reasonably suspect that they weren't dealing with a flu virus. On the other hand, they were still completely in the dark about what it actually was.

* * *

While Yuen, Peiris, and their colleagues were puzzling over this quandary, which was becoming more urgent by the day, Dr. Carlo Urbani was calling GOARN in to Viet Nam, also suspecting an avian flu variant. Urbani put the mysterious pathogen on the world agenda, and for perhaps the first time in history the world worked against a new pathogen together.

In Geneva, Dr. David Heymann knew that the new disease organism needed to be identified with the utmost speed. He also knew that he didn't have the resources at the WHO to carry out the job. He realized, in fact, that the challenge and the urgency were so great that it couldn't be left either to any one lab or institution, or to all the world's microbiologists each working with partial information, not knowing what their colleagues and rivals were up to, and constantly reinventing the wheel.

The answer, the WHO team decided, was to continue what we have called the Heymann Doctrine and create a network of collaborating experts. They would recruit a manageable number of top-level labs and help them work together, like a global version of the team of physicists working on the Manhattan Project. Most of the pieces—the labs, the researchers, the means of getting new information out to the scientific community—were in place already, but they were separate and, indeed, competitive. The vision and energy needed to combine these players and forces was exactly equal to what the WHO, with Heymann's direction, could assign to it. All it took was one person working every hour of the day and night, a person with a strong scientific background and infinite tact and patience, to pull it all together. His name was Dr. Klaus Stohr.

Over the phone Stohr speaks clearly and humbly in precise English, occasionally inventing a word that doesn't exist in English but ought to; his scientific exposition broken now and then with unexpected flashes of warmth and humor.

"We are not the ones who wanted to sit in the driver's seat. We felt ourselves as being facilitators. We were sure we had to create an atmosphere that everyone wanted to work in, and that atmosphere was not one of leadership and dominance but of... egality, of openness, of inclusiveness, of transparency."

What they created, Stohr said, was "a tailor-made system to accomplish a task. The task was to identify the pathogen which was causing the disease. From the beginning we knew that this required the resources of more than one laboratory." It required access to samples, access to certain technologies, and "the means to share the information quickly—both with those collaborating in the research and with the general medical community fighting the outbreak."

Everything began with the samples. The U.S. CDC had people on the ground in Viet Nam as part of the WHO team there, so they took samples themselves and sent them back to Atlanta. The WHO team also sent samples to the National Institute for Infectious Diseases in Japan, in the hope that this would get lab work going more quickly. It did, although the process still took two weeks, including an unfortunate incident in which a shipment of samples sat in full sunlight at Japan's Narita Airport for four days and, not surprisingly, was ruined.

Virus samples have to be packed according to the requirements of the International Postal Union, which is understandably nervous about having postal employees and the environment infected by pathogens in transit. The samples had to be packed in double containers with cotton between the containers to absorb liquid in case of a leak, and the entire assembly packed in a metal container. "And then we hope that it's being cooled," Stohr said with a kind of wary optimism. "Sometimes it's not, and then you get samples that are very well protected, but not cooled, and then there's nothing in them anymore."

The WHO was in the privileged position of knowing which labs had which samples, and this became the first criterion for inclusion in the network. The second was a willingness to take part—after all, as Stohr said candidly, some labs might have had bad experiences in working with the WHO in the past. The third was any special technical capabilities the lab might have.

One of those was special in an unexpected way.

"We were almost certain we were dealing with a new pathogen, so I wanted to have an outstanding scientist and research manager on board who had non-human primates, and he could practically set up everything within ten days." This was Dr. Albert Osterhaus of Erasmus University in Rotterdam. "By that time we already had a suspect, which he could then put immediately into the monkeys. Without this it would have taken another month, at least, to kick things off."

Osterhaus's lab at Erasmus University was the only network member that didn't already have samples of the virus ("He had great monkeys, but no samples"), but this defect was remedied in dramatic fashion. The Institut Pasteur of Paris also had representatives in Viet Nam, who shuttled samples back to France with them. There, the WHO quickly arranged for Pasteur to make samples available to Osterhaus, who had sent a car which crossed northern Europe in the darkness with its cargo of virus, delivering it to Rotterdam.

Setting up the lab network took place over one weekend. On Saturday morning, March 15, the WHO team worked out the criteria for inclusion and the rules for cooperation, and identified labs in Canada, France, Germany, Hong Kong, Japan, the Netherlands, Singapore, the United Kingdom, and the United States. (Two labs in China joined the network in early April when research results from China became internationally available.) On Sunday morning phone calls went out to representatives of each lab, and then an inventory form was sent out to find out from each lab what samples they had, what results they had already obtained, what technologies they were planning to use, and so on—all of which was immediately put up on a secure web site, the internet equivalent of the communal whiteboard. "On Monday we had the first teleconference with all of them on board."

The alliance was announced with considerable fanfare. James Hughes, director of the U.S. National Center for Infectious Diseases in Atlanta, called it "historic." "[By collaborating] we're marching two or three times faster," agreed Osterhaus.

For the next four weeks they had 60-90 minute teleconferences every day except Sundays. Stohr began each one with "Good morning, good day, good evening"—a greeting demonstrating his awareness that people across the globe were trying to mesh their schedules in the name of solving this crisis, but also alluding to the apparently endless day/night of work that everyone remembers who was submerged in the struggle against SARS.

What Stohr's own role required, he said, was "collaborative transparency and openness"—in other words, a vast amount of resolving confusions, disputes, misunderstandings, and tensions, trying to be what he called a "lubrificant" in the gearbox of the network. He is too tactful to specify, but the background was obvious: there were major reputations and egos at stake, and the line between collaboration and competition was frequently invisible.

"There were times when members feared they might be deprived of unique possibilities for scientific progress. All of them are outstanding and extraordinarily competitive individuals. Some might become Nobel prize winners. Part of science has always involved guarding one's academic cutting-edge benefits," Stohr recalled. He had anticipated this, and made sure that in the relatively light framework of rules for collaboration there were agreements to cover sharing samples and information. "We did not always succeed, but most of the time I think we could help."

Heymann and Rodier both describe Stohr as having the patience of a saint. He responded with predictable modesty.

"We are all individuals, and we all have our own plans and our own interests, and everyone's interests are equally valid. We have not to change people's interests but—perhaps—to expand them."

Above all, he said, it was a challenge in management—and he described a scenario that in some respect perfectly illustrates the Heymann Doctrine.

"We had a huge whiteboard covered with drawings so we knew who was going to have what, what the next steps would be. It was a chess game. You have to anticipate all the moves, and you had to make certain moves in order to cause others to do certain things... it was a very complex networking undertaking, but very interesting because you have some uncertainties in there, you have the subjective factors of people. What helped us was the clear understanding that we had to deliver. It was no good filling in a piece of paper at the end saying it didn't work out. We wanted to deliver. We wanted to get a result."

In order to disseminate the network's discoveries, Stohr set up another delicate bridging exercise—in this case concerning the all-important and career-making relationship between the scientists and the scientific journals.

On the one hand, the scientists wanted to see their work published under their own names in the top peer-reviewed journals, an outcome of great importance. On the other hand, the WHO wanted to get the gist of the information out to the public health community at once so it could be useful in the state of crisis. ("We said to them, 'What you have found, we have to use today. Tonight.'") The process of peer review and editing, however, can take months and normally, these journals refuse to publish research that has already been made public by other means. Stohr mentioned some of the major journals—*Nature*, *The Lancet*, *Science*, the *New England Journal of Medicine*—with whom he felt "a win-win situation" could be reached: he would help funnel the research to them if they would agree to let the WHO put the findings on its website as soon as they emerged. By this arrangement, the journals forsook the right of first publication, but by taking part in the hunt for the pathogen they were contributing to the public good, and were also publishing breaking news—an unprecedented move, and an exciting prospect.

"I must say, we had extremely positive responses and support from the journals. They understood what this was all about, and with the help of new publication technology and an expedited review process the publications were out in sometimes less than two weeks." The journals also saw what might be called the CNN Benefit: by publishing news as it was happening, they became the center of attention. One editor told Stohr that his journal had had half a million hits in a day, far more than it had ever known before.

It's perhaps the best illustration of Stohr's view of his role in the virtual network—and perhaps also of his character—that when he wrote an article for Lancet explaining how the network was set up, he went against the wishes of the network labs and the journal and removed his own name from the article prior to publication.

* * *

Back in Hong Kong, Yuen's team was now working under the intense pressure of being in the middle of the outbreak. It was a small team to begin with, roughly a dozen people, and several had clinical duties in the hospital in addition to their research work. Peiris was regularly summoned to ministerial meetings, and was working seventeen-hour days.

Nevertheless, the team had been given another opportunity to culture the new pathogen. Four days after Liu died, his brother-in-law was admitted to Kwong Wah Hospital, already severely ill. He died soon afterwards.

"This time we were smarter," Yuen said. "We did a lung biopsy."

Yuen and his team now had a section of lung tissue rich with active virus. Once again they tried to culture a disease organism from it, and once again, after fourteen days, nothing had happened.

"So we changed the cell line. We used a cell line called fetal rhesus monkey kidney cell line-FRhK4." In fact, they tried more or less every cell line that might possibly work. "We used a whole panel of cell lines that included this one. There was basically quite a bit of luck there," he admitted, writing LUCK on the board and circling it.

Luck, and some intelligent guesswork. They now knew it probably wasn't a bacterium, as patients didn't respond to antibiotics. It probably wasn't one of the well-known influenza viruses, because that avenue had been well tested and because patients didn't respond to the antiviral Tamiflu. It probably wasn't respiratory anthrax, as anthrax is easy to culture, and they would have found it already. That still left several other families of virus, though, and there was always the frightening possibility that they were facing an entirely new family of virus or an entirely new kind of pathogen, like the prions that have been proposed to account for BSE, or mad cow disease.

On March 18, a new layer of pressure was added: a lab in Germany and a different lab in Hong Kong both announced that they had found a suspect virus in blood samples from SARS patients: a paramyxovirus, a member of the same family as the virus that causes measles. The immediate response from the scientific community was cautious, but it was a plausible answer, given that pneumonia can be a complication of measles.

Nevertheless, Yuen's team decided to push on with their work. At the very least, the result needed to be confirmed, and it was always possible that even though there was paramyxovirus present in SARS patients, it was not the actual cause of the disease, or perhaps it was a kind of catalyst, helping a different virus to become more virulent.

At this point, Dr. Kwok Hung Chan takes over the story. His job was to set up and observe the cell lines—a task that kept him in the lab from 9:00 a.m. until midnight, wearing full protective equipment: this was a deadly virus with a track record of killing those in the medical profession.

When Peiris and Yuen suggested using different cell lines to grow up the virus, Chan chose half-a-dozen standard cell lines and a couple of rare cell lines, one of which was the FRhK4 cell. "Many years ago, actually, I used this cell line to grow up another virus for a study." He chuckled self-deprecatingly. "It was just an attempt. I didn't know what the outcome would be, although it was known that most monkey kidney cell lines can grow up respiratory viruses."

The test cells were kept in deep refrigeration, cooled with liquid nitrogen to minus 196 degrees Celsius. ("At this temperature, the cell can keep for years.") Chan and his assistant took out some frozen FRhK4 cells, thawed them out to resuscitate them, put them in test tubes, minced the tissue samples taken from the lung biopsy into tiny pieces using a pair of scissors, put one of these fragments in with the living cells, let the cells continue to grow for several days, and examined them daily under the microscope for signs of change.

Every day, he examined between two and three hundred test tubes for the slightest signs of changes. Most of the cell lines showed no unusual signs at all. The SARS virus, it seems, is finicky, or, to put it more scientifically, tissue-specific: it grows in only a few kinds of cell, making isolation very difficult.

After two or three days' incubation, he began to notice something happening with the FRhK4 cells. They were swelling.

This was exactly what he had been hoping for. When the virus substitutes its own RNA into the reproductive mechanism of the cell, the cell stops making copies of itself and starts making copies of the virus. These are much, much smaller than the cell, and at first no change seems to be taking place, but within a day as many as a hundred thousand viruses are teeming in the cell, and after two or three days the number may be in the millions, making the cell walls bulge and swell.

It was too early to be certain, though. Any change in the cells could also be caused by toxicity in the specimen. "We were excited, but also nervous. We didn't know whether these changes were due to the virus, or some other contaminant, or the specimen toxicity."

They took infected cells and added them to healthy cells. If the cell changes had been caused by the tissue toxicity, that effect would be diluted out. Instead, the healthy cells also started to show changes, so they knew they had a live virus at work. Another day or two later, and the swollen cells began to shrink: the cell walls had ruptured, the virus had issued out in its millions, leaving the flaccid, empty shell of the host cell.

There was still a lot of work to do. They had to examine the samples to extract the virus that had been killing the cells. They had to identify the virus, which, as the world now knows, turned out to be an entirely new coronavirus. (It was originally so named because under the electron microscope it appears to be surrounded by a ring of spikes like the circlet of a crown-corona, in Latin, meaning crown. The coronavirus family includes human common cold viruses.) The team also had to establish that it didn't fit into any of the existing three groups of coronaviruses.

They ran Polymerase Chain Reaction (PCR) tests, by which fragments of DNA can be made to replicate very rapidly and amplify a single DNA molecule into many billions of molecules. PCR can take a small sample of DNA, such as might be found on a bloody glove at a crime scene, and produce sufficient copies to carry out forensic tests.

They ran serology tests with samples of blood from recovering SARS patients to see whether the antibody their blood contained corresponded to the virus they had found.

"All these worked," Chan said. "They showed we had a single, new virus."

"The credit should go to the whole team," Yuen emphasized, writing names on the board. "Guan Yi and Zheng Bo-Jian went to Guangzhou. They risked their lives. Malik Peiris was the chief of virology supervising the virology laboratory all the time. Dr. KH Chan was the one who looked at the cell culture every day, every day, every day. He's the first person who saw the cells breaking down, dying. Leo Poon was the one who fished out the first segment of gene from the virus, who showed that this is a completely distinct virus. So it was all teamwork. I think we are the Dream Team of Hong Kong University," he finished, tongue in cheek.

* * *

Events from that moment onward, though, illustrate that the international collaboration to find the cause of SARS was less selfless and more competitive than one might wish. According to an account published in *Science*, Peiris had to attend an evening meeting of governmental advisers and missed the daily WHO SARS network phone conference on Friday, March 21. Instead, he emailed group members that he had isolated a virus from patient tissues that grew more slowly when exposed to blood serum from patients recovering from a SARS infection, he said, suggesting they had developed antibodies to the virus, while serum from healthy controls had no effect on the virus. An initial electron microscope image, he said, suggested a coronavirus.

The CDC's Respiratory and Enteric Viruses Branch was also closing in on the coronavirus, and said so on the March 21 conference call. At the same time, a trio of collaborating European groups was making similar progress, and announced during the Monday, March 24 conference call that they too were close to identifying what seemed to be a novel coronavirus. The virtual network collaboration seemed to be paying off.

Later that day, continued *Science*, when it was nighttime in Hong Kong, CDC issued a press release: "CDC Lab Analysis Suggests New Coronavirus May Cause SARS." It read, "The Centers for Disease Control and Prevention (CDC) announced today that a previously unrecognized virus from the coronavirus family is the leading hypothesis for the cause of severe acute respiratory syndrome (SARS)." The

WHO lab network was mentioned briefly; the University of Hong Kong and European groups, not at all.

Over the following days, the complex situation sorted itself out in the usual ways of the professional scientific trade. Conciliatory statements were issued. Some were feted, others overlooked. Stohr himself stressed that the labs should take the credit, rather than the WHO.

The results had to be checked and confirmed, and it wasn't until April 16 that the coronavirus was finally named, with confidence, as the culprit: It was announced that in monkey experiments at the Erasmus Medical Center, researchers showed that the new coronavirus alone can cause SARS.

To this day, the presence of paramyxovirus in SARS patients is unexplained. It may play a role as a catalyst or enabler; it may not. A great deal about SARS is still unknown.

Exactly a year later, when I visited a number of the SARS outbreak sites, it was clear that for all the talk of cooperation there was clearly a fair amount of science as usual. For many, the race had been against other institutions as much as against the outbreak. One eminent scientist chortled with glee when saying that two of his rivals had "got it wrong." Two spoke with chagrin about the fact that their teams were working against others that were larger and wealthier. Someone complained of not being able to get samples to study.

Department heads got their names published first in the list of authors of an article even though it was their juniors or their graduate students who worked 15-hour shifts. People still knew the day, time, and circumstances under which they had uploaded their data, still acutely aware that those hours or even minutes meant the difference between merely doing a good job and winning the race, between having a letter published in one of the journals as opposed to the lead article; between satisfaction and glory.

* * *

Once SARS had been identified a new race took over: a race to sequence the virus and lay its genetic structure and history bare.

Even the relatively safe process of sequencing the virus was fraught with problems. Early in the outbreak, Professor Mary Waye of the Chinese University of Hong Kong found herself at regular meetings with clinicians battling the disease (the Prince of Wales Hospital is the teaching hospital for Chinese University), but to her surprise nobody brought up the subject of asking her lab to sequence the virus. She felt an increasing sense of urgency and of wanting to do something, and in the elevator afterwards, she would say things like "We should just shotgun clone and sequence everything and see if we can find out what it is," but when she did, people would just look at her blankly. "In the medical profession, you don't do anything until it's been well tested. They usually buy tests from companies. They're not used to something that's completely new."

Waye is short, maternally plump, and speaks softly and intelligently in excellent English, as befits someone trained as a post-doctoral fellow at Cambridge. She herself had an unpleasantly close brush with the disease in mid-March, when she and several colleagues flew to a meeting in Beijing. "We weren't too concerned, but in retrospect we should have been. The flight the day before had a SARS patient on it."

When they returned, she and her colleague Stephen Tsui were asked if they'd like to try sequencing the virus. They called the lab together and asked for volunteers to work on the virus, because of the risk involved. She herself thought the risk to be slight, but others were less sanguine. Some students wanted to help, but not to work on the virus. Lab technicians and teaching assistants were uneasy. At this point the university was closed to undergraduates (the schools, too, were closed), but graduate students were still coming in. She explained that the virus would be inactivated before it left the Prince of Wales Hospital, but some were uneasy. What if it wasn't completely inactivated? What if one particle of virus in a million survived?

They worked out a safety procedure. The inactivated virus, in a test tube, was packed in ice, then put in a secure container. The courier from the Prince of Wales Hospital would bring it up the hill to Chinese University and leave it on top of a garbage container outside the back door of the seventh floor, so nobody from the lab had to meet the courier in case the courier was infected. A corridor was reserved for moving the virus to the lab.

Once the virus was in the lab, the lab was divided into "clean" and "dirty" halves, like the teams working in hospitals. Each had its own entrance. The dirty team came in their door and worked on the sequencing; the clean team handled phone calls and brought in lunches, passing them over a partition. The whole area was taped off from the public, and anyone wanting to enter had to pass a station where they signed in and wrote down contact information, donned mask, gloves, disposable gowns, protective footwear, and shower caps.

"In retrospect, all this was unnecessary, but some of our technicians and our safety coordinator were very concerned, so I wanted to placate them."

The students worked in two shifts, 24 hours a day, on the sequencing. Three were due to graduate, but put off finishing their graduate work to work on SARS. The lab was also low on reagents necessary for sequencing the SARS virus, and had no grant money to buy any. "I said to Stephen, 'I have a car, you have a car—if necessary, we'll sell our cars.'" They ended up spending more than HK$20,000, hoping it would somehow be repaid.

"It was exhausting," she said from the bottom of her heart. It wasn't just the lab work that took so much time and energy. Simply keeping pace with the crisis was a full-time job. They had to constantly read papers and web pages for breaking information. The university had meetings all the time to address questions that had never arisen before. What do you do when a medical student becomes infected? Medical students live in dorms—what happens when an infected student has just thrown a party? Do you quarantine everyone who was at the party? How do you handle the classes that have been suspended? The faculty were supposed to teach by web, but that in turn involved transferring vast amounts of teaching materials and notes to the web, and then answering a constant flow of student emails.

On Sunday, April 13, Waye and her husband went for a hike on the Peak in Hong Kong. Coincidentally, Fred Leung, whose lab was also working on the sequencing, was doing exactly the same, with his wife: the government had recommended that everyone get as fit as possible to build up their immunity in case they contracted the virus. Both parties' cell phones rang at almost the same moment: both were being called to let them know that a team of researchers at the British Columbia Cancer Research Centre in Vancouver had sequenced the virus' genome and had posted the sequence on the Web. Both Waye and Leung rushed back to their labs to see the results; both were crushed that they had been beaten by only a day or two; both made the observation that the Canadian group had been given a sample a good two weeks before their own labs. Both talked to their teams and raised their spirits and put the issue to a vote; both teams decided to keep going, to confirm the Canadian result, if nothing else. "A bit of redundancy doesn't hurt," Waye said philosophically. "The better we know the virus, the better we can detect it."

* * *

What did the sequencing show? Apart from confirming that it was indeed a new coronavirus, the genome gave some fascinating clues about the history and evolution of the virus, its viral genealogy. Specimens taken from all over the world demonstrated clearly that these virus specimens were indeed all descendants of the one transported by Dr. Liu. Samples taken from Dr. Liu's brother-in-law produced a surprise: "In [him] we picked up two genotypes," said Fred Leung. "Two genotypes. That means two things. First, the virus was mutating very fast. Second, it will pose a very difficult challenge to develop a vaccine." It might have mutated in the brother-in-law; or he might have been co-infected from someone else.

The SARS virus genome showed a very strong similarity to the one from the coronavirus later found in the Himalayan masked palm civet and other exotic wildlife found in the live-animal markets of South China, adding further circumstantial evidence suggesting that the markets were involved in the chain of transmission, with certain sections seeming avian in origin.

"We think that the civet cat is actually an intermediate host, not the origin of the animal source," said Fred Leung. "Still at this point we don't know the animal reservoir for SARS. We think that it may even be of avian origin, but unfortunately nobody has found any SARS coronavirus in birds." Perhaps chickens were involved after all.

* * *

At the same time as the virtual lab network was making spectacular progress in identifying and characterizing the virus, two other virtual networks had been set up by the WHO and were working on allied subjects, and it may be instructive to compare their success.

One was a clinicians' group, run by Dr. Mark Salter, seconded from the United Kingdom. The other was an epidemiology-and-surveillance group led by Dr. Angela Merianos, on loan from Australia, that was culling the incoming information from different countries and trying to work out the incubation period, the rate of infection, trying to set up mathematical models that would predict best- and worse-case scenarios for the rate of spread.

All three did excellent work under stressful conditions; all three produced a series of scientific papers. By most accounts, though, the virtual network of laboratories was by far the most successful of the three. Clinicians interviewed in several countries didn't mention the WHO virtual network at all as a resource, and seem to have focused their attention much closer to home. Some physicians called friends and colleagues in other countries for advice, but these connections were few, and were limited to those in senior positions. Those on the front lines lacked the connections, and in any case were far too busy.

Barbara Yaffe, the Toronto Public Health Incident Manager, recalled somewhat testily: "We could have spent all our day doing teleconferences but we were too busy fighting fires. We were killing ourselves fighting this thing."

"One of the ingredients for success," Stohr reflected, "is that you have to have a common target. You have to have a relatively narrow focus. So from that perspective the work in this network was easier to organize. What also helped was this "lubrification," this bringing people together and making sure that their particular private individual needs and concerns were being addressed," which would have been impossible if the network had consisted of fifty or even more people.

"Another reason was that we had a scientific task to fulfill, and we had scientists on board. With clinicians, who work in a hospital, their daily priorities are driven by the needs of their patients. Many but not all have necessarily a very strong scientific background. Not all of them have been intimately involved in setting up clinical trials and sharing data in international research projects. The approaches chosen by the clinicians were based on an emergency intervention. It was a new disease, nothing worked, so what clinicians do is they try things out and see what works best."

Different physicians tried different treatments, he went on, but often under differing circumstances for a small number of patients. How could the results be compared, especially with such small sample sizes? "For us it was easier because the laboratory methods are not so different. Comparing clinical data is much more difficult, much more complicated."

Similar problems of scope and scale also made the work of the epidemiological network immensely hard.

"For epidemiological conclusions you have to have a good sample size, you have to have a well designed study protocol, and you have to bring together the laboratory and the epi data. How can you deduce the transmissibility of a virus not knowing how long it's been excreted? You won't know the excretion duration and the excretion patterns and how much is excreted by which excreta and secreta if no one has taken samples from these patients and if no one has used the proper laboratory technology on these samples. In the end you can compare these laboratory results with the epidemiological observations of how many people have been infected during which stage of the disease. Bringing this all together is a very complex undertaking which depends on many, many variables ... many of them are new, are unknown, can change quickly, disappear, and new factors can come in... "

Which perhaps begins to explain why there are still unexplained transmissions of the virus, and why at times it seems to have behaved so capriciously, with Patient A showing full-fledged symptoms but infecting nobody and Patient B showing very mild symptoms and infecting sixteen people in less than an hour.

Two final observations about the virtual networks:

First, even when they were only partly successful in terms of generating new real-time practical information, they were helping to advance our understanding of the virus at a greatly accelerated rate, and generating research that may turn out to be valuable even if it didn't emerge until long after the outbreak was over.

Second, their virtuality was a strength but also a limitation. One of the most deeply-felt sentiments about the outbreak was from Dr. Bonnie Henry, who in late May and early June visited the outbreak sites in Taiwan, Hong Kong, and Beijing on a fact-finding tour with three other officials from Toronto Public Health. What struck her and everyone she met, she said, was how similar the outbreak was in all these diverse settings; and how the people in each place had the same sense of being shunned by the rest of the world—in her words, a pariah state. She wished that she and her colleagues could have been visited by representatives of the WHO so the world body could really grasp what was going on—and so that those fighting SARS might feel less isolated and alone.

Virtual networks, if clearly focused, probably have their place, and will probably continue to be used; but as with the basic business of treating a sick patient, a besieged health care force also needs a good dose of human company.

* * *

"In the 1980s, it took 2 years to identify HIV as the cause of AIDS," wrote Barry Bloom, the Dean of the Harvard School of Public Health. "In 2003, WHO created an extraordinary network of 13 laboratories in 10 countries... which identified a virus associated with SARS in 2 weeks and had its entire genome sequenced in 2 more. Those labs shared their knowledge in an unprecedented fashion, to the benefit of everyone."

While this is true, it could also be said that, in a curious way, the winner of the race was the virus. Identifying it did little more than throw a kind of spotlight on it, magnifying it from the invisible to the visible. It became a star of the emerging infectious disease circuit.

It also kept much of its mystery—a masked creature, like its human hosts. Despite the astonishing amount of scientific work achieved at unprecedented speed, we still know very little that will do us a great deal of good in the future. We don't know, for example, what will become of SARS. Some viruses adapt to their human hosts and lose virulence over successive generations; some become more dangerous, either increasing in virulence or becoming more efficient at spreading from person to person.

"SARS is still around," said Paul Tam of the University of Hong Kong. "It is lurking in the background. It's still out there. It may not be the same SARS but it may be SARS 2. It may be SARS 3. It can always come back."

The viral archaeology gives little more than a series of fascinating but inconclusive hints about the origins and by implications the hidden whereabouts of the virus. Moreover, the SARS coronavirus is so hard to work with—and therefore so expensive—that some experts in the field have predicted that, unless there is another significant outbreak, funding for research into vaccines and anti-viral treatments may dry up within a year.

If that turns out to be true—and we have yet to see that galvanizing outbreak—it's possible that the SARS coronavirus will have put in a short, devastating cameo appearance on the planet, disappearing as mysteriously as it arrived, leaving little more in its wake than some sequences in GenBank, a few dozen scientific papers, and an electron microscope photograph of a crown of thorns.

Chapter 12.

One Deep: A Case Study in Public Health in Toronto

O At 10:00 a.m. on March 13, 2003, Linda Davis, an infection control practitioner at the Scarborough Hospital (Grace Division)—a title universally abbreviated to "Scarborough Grace"—called Carola Ostach, a Toronto Public Health inspector specializing in infectious diseases and said, "The TB smear came back negative. Do you think it's possible this has something to do with what's happening in Hong Kong?"

SARS caused a public health crisis everywhere, but the city of Toronto saw probably the most developed and extensive public health effort to contain the disease-an effort that showed how critical the public health system is in times of an outbreak of infectious disease, yet how even in a major western nation an outbreak can bring this system to the brink of collapse.

By the time Davis called Ostach, Toronto Public Health (TPH) had, unwittingly, already been constructively involved in the outbreak for several days. The case in question was a 43-year-old man we'll call Mr. Qin, whose mother had fallen ill after returning from Hong Kong. She had seen a family physician who had diagnosed—correctly, as it turned out—an unspecified virus, but she died at home in the early hours of March 5th without ever being admitted to a hospital. Qin had been admitted to hospital on March 7 suffering from a non-specific but severe respiratory complaint. The hospital suspected tuberculosis: the city of Toronto sees several hundred cases each year, many brought back by residents and immigrants from areas of the world where tuberculosis is still endemic. TPH was alerted, as per the protocol required in the case of tuberculosis or several other "notifiable" communicable diseases. (While any communicable disease is by definition a potential public health problem, not all public health systems respond in the same ways to, nor have the same criteria for, these notifiable diseases.) The TB team had taken specimens and tested them, but the results had just come back negative. When the hospital heard that the mother had recently died at home (supposedly of heart failure), danger signals went off, and Davis called Ostach.

The virus was also moving quickly: the son's disease progressed at a speed that astonished the hospital, and he died the same afternoon. "The physician was stunned and distraught," Ostach said. "He kept saying, `Is there anything else I could have done? What did I miss?'"

Ironically, the speed of the public health response turned out to have its own dangers. The TB team had already begun the process of contact tracing, had identified the rest of the family as contacts, and had referred them to their own family doctors. The extended Qin family was already visiting those doctors, taking SARS with them.

* * *

At Scarborough Grace, it was the Prince of Wales story all over again: one day ten staff were ill, the next morning 14, with 19 infected by that evening. "Sunday was the most surreal day," said Bonnie Henry, one of the city's Associate Medical Officers of Health, as if still stunned. Short, blonde, athletic, soft-spoken, she is a person capable of great exertions when necessary: photos on the wall of her office show her running the Paris Marathon. SARS would prove to be an even greater test of endurance.

The health authority opened an old TB ward in the West Park Hospital, which had individual rooms set up with negative pressure—in other words, air was not allowed to escape the room. They then had to call all the sick nurses, X-ray technicians, and respiratory therapists and tell them, essentially, "We don't know what you have. Don't say goodbye. Don't hug your kids. Go to West Park, now, and we'll do our best."

Doing their best involved two overlapping and theoretically related activities. The hospitals would do their best, like hospitals in a score of countries, to work out how best to prevent their patients dying of pneumonia. Toronto Public Health would do its best, like public health authorities in a score of countries, to prevent the outbreak spreading throughout the population. Hospitals and doctors, the matinee stars of medicine, can treat only those who are already sick; in an epidemic they will get swamped at once unless public health can prevent others from becoming infected. In essence, this means getting the names of those who are sick and identifying everyone who might have infected them, and who they in turn may have infected.

SARS, as we've already seen, demanded a whole new layer of significance and urgency on top of this already complicated and time-consuming public health work: it demanded diagnosis by epidemiology. A hospital would call and ask, "Have you guys found the link that's going to make this person a SARS case?" Time and again it would be the presence or absence of an "epi link"—a clear and traceable contact with another SARS case—that would determine whether someone should be treated as a probable SARS patient.

While medicine by epidemiology is not seen as much in Western countries, it's not uncommon in the developing world. Individuals with diarrhea in Bangladesh during the hurricane season don't all get their stool tested; it's presumed they have cholera. In a sense, it's a Western luxury not to think in the collective fashion. To be able to treat a single patient at a time is one of the key privileges of medicine in the West. In the developing world, medicine is so dependent on public health that the two are often the same.

In Toronto, diagnosis by epidemiological detective work began at once. TPH needed to know immediately which members of the index family, the Qins, were infected, and whom they might have infected in turn. The human element in contact tracing made their job more difficult than they had imagined.

Dr. Carola Ostach is a calm, strongly-built woman who looks as if she would be best in a crisis. "The husband in the first family, [the one] who had traveled to Hong Kong?" she chuckled. "He denied ever having been to Hong Kong. Three conversations I had with him, through an AT&T interpreter—he denied having gone with his wife. He felt we were authority figures and he was going to get in trouble, and didn't tell the truth. But thank goodness, the daughter was still able to let us know that yes, indeed, he had traveled as well."

Meanwhile, Mark Bartlett, a public health inspector with a sandy moustache and the affable eagerness of a scoutmaster, was tracing in the opposite direction. He needed to find the airline that the Qins had used in order to see whether anyone on the plane had fallen sick.

Before falling ill, a family member told him that the Qins had flown on Continental, but when he called the airline, he said, Continental told him: "We don't fly to Toronto."

Bartlett was frantic. He had to get permission to enter the Qins' house, now deserted, to look not only for any clues that might tell him anything about the disease, but to see if there was anything that would tell him which airline they'd traveled on. Luckily, in the basement, he found their luggage with the tags still attached: Continental.

* * *

While all this was taking place out in the community, the main office of Toronto Public Health was being turned into the SARS Command and Control Center.

The TPH headquarters is at 277 Victoria Street in the heart of tourist Toronto, a block from the Eaton Center, opposite a square where 80,000 people demonstrated against the war in Iraq. The building is surrounded by high-rises, hotels, offices, brand-name stores, overpriced restaurants, large digital billboards, and a huge picture of Jennifer Lopez in a peignoir pushing her line of perfumes. On the outside, 277 Victoria has a briefly impressive faux-stainless-steel facade, but inside, a year after the SARS outbreak, it shows unmistakable signs of low-budget spending and recent wear and tear: small offices, small cubicles, a functioning minimum of furniture. The walls on the eighth floor are bare of decoration, covered with orphan pins and tacks, scraps of masking tape, and scars where tape has been ripped off, taking paint with it.

Like every other public health department in the world, TPH did not have a purpose-built command center ready to take on an epidemic. To their credit, TPH recognized at once that a vast enterprise was opening up with frightening speed, and at once they had a stroke of luck. Three floors of 277 Victoria had just been vacated by the Toronto Housing Corporation, and within 48 hours TPH had set up phone lines, desks, dividers, chairs, bulletin boards, and even the first few computers.

The tenth floor was dedicated to a hotline, staffed from roughly 8:00 a.m. until 11:00 p.m. by two shifts of public health nurses at roughly 40 to a shift. More than 200 staff worked on the hotline during the outbreak.

On March 14th, TPH put out a press release telling the public that there were five members of a family who were ill and two deaths that might be linked to the "atypical pneumonia" in Hong Kong. Through the media, TPH asked anyone who had been in contact with the family (including at the mother's funeral) to call. All kinds of people called: some just wanting information, some already moving down the infinitely branching paths of personal contact. My aunt got out of the hospital a week ago and my whole family had dinner with her last night. What should we do? My child goes to school with another child whose parents have SARS. What should we do?

It was so early in the outbreak, often the people staffing the hotline didn't know all the answers and had to ask their manager on duty, who might not know either.

"When people called in," Mark Bartlett explained, "there was obviously a lot of tension in their voices, a lot of anxiety. In some cases they were actually already starting to come down with symptoms. I remember one call I got from a lady whose husband had already gone to the hospital with SARS-like illness, and he was quite sick. She was at her wits' end. She was starting to come down with it herself, and she had two kids, both under the age of ten. She really should have gone to the hospital [at once] for an assessment.

"This was at eleven o'clock at night after I'd already worked sixteen hours and we were just getting ready to go home. I couldn't do anything for her. Nobody would take her kids. Her relatives wouldn't take her kids because they were concerned that her kids had it, and would pass it on to them."

If this sounds heartless, it's important to remember that at this point, so early in the outbreak, everyone who had caught the disease had died or was still in hospital. No one had got better. In Bonnie Henry's words, "It was three weeks before we knew it was a three-week disease." Even so, it was weeks more, or even months, before some recovered. One Toronto paramedic was still not back at work a year after getting sick. In retrospect, SARS may seem like a bad pneumonia; through mid-April 2003, in many people's minds it was still a death sentence.

"There was no agency that would take the kids," Bartlett went on, agitated. "They weren't sick, so technically they couldn't go into a hospital, and so this lady had no options.

"I left it with her: 'Listen, if you get so sick during the night that you get highly acute, call, get an ambulance and they'll find something to do with your kids.'"

That was more or less what happened. The mother did end up in the hospital, and TPH arranged for the Hospital for Sick Children to take and look after her two children, give them bed space, and let them live there.

"It was terrible, because in public health, most of the time when you intervene you're able to do something positive to help, but here it was like, 'I can't do anything. There's nothing I can do that's going to help this woman.' I got off the phone and just stared into space, going 'What the hell's happening here?' It was just awful."

This went on for three months. By June 24, the hotline had taken more than 300,000 calls—as many as 47,567 in a single day.

Geri Nephew was drafted in as a hotline manager: "There were days when calls were coming in so fast you couldn't even hang up the phone. As soon as a client would hang up, the next call would pop in."

The ninth floor was for contact follow-up. In all, 13,374 people were placed in quarantine, almost all of them voluntarily, and every person in quarantine had to be called twice every day, ideally, to take down their most recent temperature check, to ask about symptoms, to arrange food deliveries if necessary, to offer mental health counseling if necessary, and frankly to make sure they were at home. The contact tracers were, in a sense, the unguarded border between health and sickness. Quarantine relied largely on people's willingness to comply, and the public health nurse's ability to convey both sympathy and a sense of civic responsibility was an important factor in sustaining people's patience at a very tough time.

Ingenuity and perseverance in contact tracing and follow-up became essential whenever there was a contact nexus—a person or site where many people might have been infected. Bartlett had to get hold of a doctor who was on vacation on a Caribbean cruise. "He had been exposed, and we didn't know if he was enjoying his cruise or sitting in sick bay." (Not to mention the possibility that the cruise ship was spreading SARS around the Caribbean.) They urgently needed his medical records to do contact tracing, but his office was locked. Guessing that someone would be checking on his house and watering his plants, they left a message on his front door asking for a phone call—a ploy that turned out to be successful, though TPH had arranged with the Toronto police to break into the office if necessary.

The eighth floor was charged with case management—in other words, keeping track of every confirmed or suspected SARS patient, whether in hospital or at home under quarantine.

"Referrals were flooding in so fast we had to set up a special physician reporting line," Geri Nephew said. "We ended up having to install a special administrators' phone line as well, where hospital administrators could contact us... all of our cell phones would be bombarded as soon as people got hold of the manager's phone number. Our pagers would be full, our cell phones would be full. You couldn't respond fast enough." Some 2,000 patients were followed in this detailed fashion, with every change of health or status tracked. Each of these investigations took an average of nine hours, and likely involved other contacts and other possible cases.

"One lady was intubated," Ostach said, "and as she was being intubated she got out, 'Old man going to nursing home.' That was all we had. The hospital phoned me and said, 'I don't know how you're going to pull this one off, but this guy's going to a nursing home, he's a contact of someone who's very, very ill. Good luck!'

"I thought, 'How am I going to find this guy?' Luckily we have a system set up where there's an organization called CCAC (Community Care Access Centre), and they're the ones who farm people out [to nursing homes]. They have lists of people who want to be placed somewhere. Thank God, it was a man, because most of the people in nursing homes are female. So I decided to call CCAC, tell them that he's going somewhere today, and maybe they can find him. I had the lady's address of where she came from, in hopes that they were living together." They were able to track him down actually in the van en route. "He was on the way to a nursing home, and they were able to pull him back."

But even then, the situation posed problems. "He was unable to care for himself, and nobody wanted to take him. The lady in the hospital was actually his nurse, who lived in with him in this apartment. So that was when the province let us use a nursing home, outside of Toronto, that hadn't yet been opened, just for SARS contacts who were elderly."

* * *

Transport of SARS patients or suspects was one of the most hazardous and critically important aspects of the entire operation. If trained physicians in hospitals had difficulty diagnosing SARS patients among a patient population that had already been triaged two or three times, imagine the job facing a paramedic called to the bedroom of an elderly woman, about whom the only information was that she was having trouble breathing. It could be cardiac problems, asthma, anxiety, emphysema... or SARS. And instead of simply examining the patient, the paramedic would have to get her onto a stretcher and through the twists and turns of furniture and stairs—what Peter Macintyre, manager of Community Safeguard Services for Toronto Emergency Medical Services, called "uncontrolled environments"—performing any number of awkward movements that might dislodge a mask. All paramedics were ordered to wear full PPE from March 28th on—and ordered to shave too, to ensure a better fit.

If those were the hazardous jobs (three paramedics and a supervisor developed mild SARS), the critical jobs were hospital-to-hospital transfers. The two principal ways in which SARS spread were by infecting people within a hospital, and then by traveling with those people when they went to other hospitals. Toronto EMS, already taking more than 400 emergency calls a day, was given control over all the private operators who do most hospital transfers, and set up an operations center that ensured nobody was moved anywhere without preliminary triage, a questionnaire, and the signature of a physician if there was the remotest possibility of SARS.

If EMS services were under such strain even with the centralized system that Toronto had quickly set up, Macintyre pointed out, how would a city like New York manage, with seventy-five hospitals, each with its own ambulance service, and numerous private operators? "How are you going to control that? That's a big challenge."

* * *

Toronto Public Health discovered quite quickly what the rest of the affected areas were experiencing: that a medical epidemic causes an information epidemic.

TPH started using an Excel spreadsheet to keep track of cases, but it was quickly overwhelmed.

"As this thing grew exponentially," Barbara Yaffe said, "we did not have an information system that could handle the information properly. We were using paper records and Post-It notes. It was completely ridiculous. One senior manager was sitting just counting numbers until 3 a.m. because there was no information system."

They called in computing assistance and began developing the Case and Contact Management System (CCMS)—a software package other countries have since used as well—but it was a constant work-in-progress, and was incompatible with the province's existing system.

"We were building the bucket," said Bonnie Henry wryly, "while we were fighting the fire."

One of the main problems for the tenth floor, which housed the hotline workers, was how to provide information that was both accurate and consistent. The answer was binders. Useful phone numbers (the Salvation Army and Red Cross food lines, the neighboring health units, EMS, Health Canada, the numbers of medical professionals, and dozens of others), FAQs and protocols were gathered by the floor managers and compiled in ring binders updated daily by Alba Eremita. Every day saw new information, added, or changed pages: Eremita had to come in early, type up the new sheets, put them in plastic binder pockets and get at least one binder ready for the manager by the beginning of the morning briefing, and by the time the briefing ended she had to have an updated binder by every phone.

While the tenth floor was drowning in questions, the ninth floor was asking questions and drowning in answers. Just one of the details that needed to be tracked, for example, was requests for masks and thermometers. Five masks a day was the recommended supply; every time a mask got wet, taken off, or otherwise touched by hand, it was supposed to be replaced. TPH developed an assembly line: the public health nurse wrote up a phone order for masks and/or thermometers and dropped it in a pick-up box. Every 30-45 minutes a clerical worker circulated through that floor, picked up the completed orders, and took them to Sherine Bento. She entered the details into the database and faxed the forms to the courier—usually volunteers from the Red Cross or the Salvation Army, but sometimes even the Toronto Public Library system, as it has a home delivery service for books. The courier made the delivery and faxed a confirmation, which Bento also entered into the database. Any given day might involve as many as 100 orders; each order might include as many as 120 masks.

The eighth floor's paper blizzard was notable for patients' files, which created not only problems in keeping track of files, but a massive confidentiality issue. At first files went missing or got accidentally duplicated. After awhile one locked room was devoted to the files. Only a manager could open it in the morning, and retrieve the files needed for the day. During the day a file might be updated three or more times as the patient was called or his or her condition changed. At the end of the day, all the files had to be assembled, organized, and locked away.

Given that this was diagnosis by epidemiology and pandemic control by containment, everyone was important. The health care system was no longer a hierarchy with the doctors at the top, though the doctors were certainly at greater risk than some of the others. The clerical workers who got the mask orders out were an essential part of the containment team—in fact, members of the community who stayed at home and obeyed their quarantine order were also playing a critical part in containing the outbreak. This was public health at its most public: it showed how profoundly the actions of one are responsible for the health of all.

* * *

It quickly became clear that TPH needed to have someone in each hospital to keep questions and information flowing back and forth between the two sister branches of health care. As with so much else, this was a job description that had to be invented, a job that had to be carried out by someone drafted from elsewhere.

"It was sort of scary," said Karietha Cooke in her faint Caribbean accent. "I was coming out of family health where I'm dealing with babies and new moms. I was given a pager and told, 'Go!' You learned as you went."

She was sent to Sunnybrook Hospital and set up in the infection control practitioners' office, a room perhaps ten feet by twenty that was already being used by three full-time infection control practitioners and one part-timer, an absurdly small number for such a large hospital. All of them felt strongly that if their job had been taken more seriously and given a higher priority, the outbreak might not have happened. (Scarborough had one infection control practitioner for each of its two hospitals.)

Cooke's job was to interview SARS patients to try to find out where they had been in the last ten days, whom they had seen, what public places, restaurants, events they had visited. If they had been to a funeral, TPH would need to contact the funeral director and get a list of everyone present. All that contact information then had to be faxed back to Victoria Street to the case manager.

"As a nurse, you're trained to make the person feel comfortable and not seem afraid because then you'll make them feel afraid. The first time I went in, I was afraid. Deep down you're thinking, 'Oh my God, get me out of this room right away.'"

Let's spell this out: this was a potentially fatal disease communicated by close proximity. Cooke's job was to get close enough to hear what someone with seriously impaired breathing was trying to say-through a mask.

"My first interview, I'm trying to stay calm, I'm writing and my hands are shaking. I forgot how to spell simple words. But after awhile there's a sense of duty, a sense that you've got to get the job done."

She had to wear her mask even in her office. "You can imagine the headaches people had all the time, and the sinus problems."

In the hospitals, it was easy for a public health worker to feel cut off. The unsteady flow of new information about the disease and the strategies for addressing it might have been coming into Victoria Street, but there was no mechanism for getting it out to the liaisons, who, being outsiders, were also not part of the loop at the hospital either.

"Decisions would be made but you wouldn't know about them for days." A good example was personal protective equipment, or PPE. "At first I just went in with a mask. After awhile we realized we needed N95 masks, gloves and gowns." This was easier said than done, as the N95 masks had to be fit-tested so they conformed to the contours of the individual's face. "After working in the hospital for a couple of months you realized you were wearing the wrong mask all along."

* * *

In theory, the hospital liaisons were providing crucial data that would be recorded, processed, and disseminated by the TPH epidemiologists at 277 Victoria, but TPH was forced to practice what might be called crisis epidemiology.

One survivor of the SARS era is Les Shulman, a young, hip-looking guy with earring, lip beard, glasses, and a slightly stunned look. He had been on vacation, and came back in early April to find the field epidemiologists from Health Canada packing to leave, summoned by the province.

"It was really challenging. When I came back there was, like, two staff. Paper was coming at us in heaps. We had barely enough time to get all the basic information in—whether they were in hospital, whether they were in ICU, whether they were on respirators, how old they were, what sex they were, how they got it—and send a report out, let alone check that all the information was accurate. It was nuts."

Epidemiology relies on a cycle: getting information, making some sense of it, reporting it, formulating or perhaps reformulating a set of questions, and going back out to get more information. That cycle was, to say the least, heavily stressed during SARS in two crucial respects.

First, the sheer volume of data needed, and flooding in, was so great that mistakes were inevitably made taking it in and recording it. The epi forms were changing on a daily basis as it became clear that new sets of questions needed to be asked. Data entry staff were also changing frequently since the heavy workload was causing or worsening migraines, nausea and elbow pain, to say nothing of stress on the eyes. The sheer fact that every case manager might use a slightly different shorthand, or would use common phrases to mean slightly different things, meant that the consistent and reliable information that is an epidemiologist's lifeblood was under duress.

There were also institutional IT weaknesses. TPH had no way of telling when a patient had visited more than one hospital—and given that a person sick with SARS might well be intubated, unable to speak, with no relatives allowed, tracing was a nightmare. "A lot of people who were in with SARS would go from one hospital to another to another," explained Karietha Cooke, "and there'd be nothing to show they'd been at Scarborough Grace."

Second, so much data were coming in that analyzing them completely or even reflecting on them was out of the question. The medical investigator or epidemiologist as detective—there just wasn't time. "The entire time, we were reactive," Shulman muttered. "We were always playing catch-up... we were often on the phone until three or four in the morning trying to clarify individual cases."

A certain rhythm developed: hotline and contact tracing calls were made during the day and the evening, but after about 11:00 or 11:30 p.m. Toronto went to bed, so there was no longer any point to making calls. The hotline staff and contact tracers went home, but now the epidemiologists had to stay up trying to pull together the day's information, correct errors, come up with numbers for the province and for the city's next-day press conference. Shulman became famous for his all-nighters; in fact, a year later he still looked tired.

Reporting was in some respects the most stressful element of all. "We had so many different audiences that the dissemination part was also a real challenge. With the Ministry, trying to negotiate the information they needed versus what we had at the time."

This was a tactful way of saying that the Ministry of Health (at the provincial level) was constantly making demands that Toronto city's public health structure could barely meet, if at all.

"At one point they said `We need to have access to everything you have. We need a daily line-list of all the probable and suspect cases. And also people who are under investigation.' On those people, especially, we often didn't have where or when they were exposed... at one point they sent people down to try to get information from our files. They were getting in our way, asking the same people the same questions. It was crazy . . . ."

In the province's defense, they had Health Canada (the national health agency) breathing down their necks, who in turn had the WHO wanting "real-time" information. If, as Bonnie Henry thinks, the WHO included Toronto in its travel advisories on the basis of outdated information, this log-jam of epidemiological information alone might have accounted for those delays.

One consulting firm estimated that by June 12 alone, the outbreak had cost Toronto $190 million in lost tourism revenues. The calculus of an outbreak is always shaky, but it's hard to avoid the suspicion that $10 million spent on a well-staffed, integrated health care data system with plenty of surge capacity would pay for itself numerous times over in the case of an epidemic.

* * *

As it happened, Toronto had far-sightedly begun work on its own elements of a national Pandemic Influenza Plan nine months before SARS struck.

At first it was hard to get people in Toronto to care about epidemic planning. Yet everyone who was persuaded to become part of the process was already several steps ahead of the game when SARS struck.

For example: The first municipal meetings on the Pandemic Plan showed a great deal about the traditions of public safety management. After all, the city, like most cities, had a history of subway fires and train derailments, but not epidemics or biohazards.

"Public health had not been high on the radar screen here," explained Bonnie Henry, "so the Chief of Police naturally assumed charge." The police had always taken charge of any emergency, including the important business of making any necessary public statements.

"Really?" Henry asked. "What if it's anthrax? What if it's smallpox?"

This gave everyone pause for thought, as did the planning process as a whole. When SARS struck, the deputy chief of police called her and asked, "Bonnie, what can we do to help?" It turned out they could do a great deal. They helped to deliver supplies to families in quarantine. On the rare occasions when Public Health had to issue an official—i.e., involuntary—order of quarantine, the police served the order. "A policeman in a mask with a gun was very effective," she chuckled.

Conversely, Henry worked with the police occupational health services to make sure that the police, too, were protected, making sure they had daily updates about the outbreak, training them on proper use of their protective equipment. When she saw a police officer outside a hospital directing traffic wearing a mask and gloves, she put in a call.

Other potential partners and stakeholders in epidemic planning were coroners and funeral directors. Days before SARS arrived, Henry had been talking to a group of funeral directors—a surprisingly engaged and jolly group, she said—who had a range of public health questions she could never have predicted. In the case of a pandemic flu outbreak, was it safe to cremate? What about Jewish funerals and sitting shiva? What if the family wanted the body shipped back to, say, Italy? How about embalming?

These questions would come back almost at once, but now as practical rather than theoretical concerns, and with great urgency and emotional weight. In Islam, washing the body after death is of great importance—yet during the SARS outbreak, it was at best impractical and probably extremely dangerous. Henry discussed the question with an imam, and reached a compromise: the family watched through glass as funeral home staff in full protective gear washed the body.

* * *

One of the most important areas for which nobody was prepared was public health law.

"We were dealing with a new disease," explained Jane Speakman, a lawyer for the city of Toronto specializing in communicable disease issues, "that wasn't considered in the [existing] legislation at all. If a communicable disease was on the list, it opened up all kinds of doors in terms of a legal response. Tuberculosis, for example. If someone had TB and they weren't taking their pills and they were infectious, there's a section in the legislation, under Section 22, which enables the Medical Officer of Health to order someone with a communicable disease to take certain steps. Quarantine would be one, but it could be as straightforward as `Put yourself under the care and treatment of a physician and follow the treatment ordered by your doctor.' For someone who is HIV-positive it would require someone to notify their partners. It wasn't always quarantine—it could be any number of community protection measures." In other words, the law could compel someone to behave in a socially responsible fashion.

"In the statute, it says that you have to meet certain conditions before you can even write the order. Communicable disease has to be present, it has to present a risk to the community, if you're going to issue an order, the order has to be necessary to decrease or eliminate the risk to the community—those three things have to be there before you can even write your order.

"SARS was not included on the list of communicable diseases. If we ever needed to take the step of asking people to quarantine themselves and also to take their temperature and report to public health, we had no legal authority to do that.

This presented two problems: SARS had to be added to the list of communicable diseases as quickly as possible, but physicians also had to supply Speakman with a list of diagnostic criteria that would determine who potentially had SARS, and thus could be issued an order.

"At the beginning, I think it's fair to say that people were working blind. They didn't know what they were dealing with. With TB, you could use an X-ray, or a skin test, or sputum samples to make a confirmed diagnosis. We didn't have those kinds of tests for SARS, but there were some pretty clear signs and symptoms."

The legislation was changed with remarkable dispatch on March 25th. (The provincial state of emergency was declared on March

22nd.) Fortunately, it involved a regulation change rather than a statute change, a simpler and easier process.

This law change not only defined SARS as a communicable disease but also as a virulent disease, which meant that health professionals were now required to report any suspected SARS cases to TPH.

"If you have a communicable disease that is also listed as a virulent disease—tuberculosis, for example—it gives you some more powers to take even more drastic action." To be specific, a civil detention can be ordered for a period of up to four months in order to protect the community. If someone were to be criminally prosecuted for violation of this legal order, he or she could also be fined as much as $5,000 a day.

"We didn't issue orders on every SARS patient; we didn't issue orders telling people they had to be quarantined. We only did it in a very few cases, and we only did it when it was absolutely urgent to do so."

Only 27 cases were deemed absolutely urgent, which was just as well: issuing legal orders for all 13,374 quarantines would have added yet more burden to the already disastrous overload of work at TPH, and would have thrown considerable additional strain on the Toronto legal system. In the vast majority of cases, a verbal order was enough.

Another significant change in the legislation allowed TPH to issue a quarantine order to a group of people, whereas before it had been set up only to allow one order to be given to one person. Issuing several hundred individual orders would have taken up absurd amounts of precious time.

In planning for issuing orders, the luxury of time didn't exist during SARS, not just because everyone was overworked, but because every hour of delay meant the possibility of several new contacts and infections.

"We felt that we had to be ready to go at a moment's notice. I had no idea what time of day or night Bonnie or one of the other associates would call me and say, `We need an order, and we need it right away.' We decided to develop templates. There were a number of different circumstances that we might be finding ourselves in, but several of the requirements in the order would be the same. So we nailed that down and came up with instructions for everybody so the Associate Medical Officers of Health could just quickly fill in the blanks." It was also important, however, to make sure extra detail was added to customize the order to fit the case, especially noting the reasons for the order: "people have to understand why you're telling them to do something."

Looking ahead, they realized that they might need to get an order quickly at a time that was inconvenient for the judge and/or the court—after all, the Easter weekend was coming up. "So we phoned the court and said, 'As you're well aware, there's an outbreak of SARS.' These are the powers that the Medical Officer of Health has. If someone breaches a Section 22, just like we would in a TB order that was breached, we would come before the court to bring our application to have the person detained. The courts made themselves available, they gave us the names of judges, we gave them copies of the legislation so they would know what was needed. They also wanted us to make sure that the individual had an opportunity to be legally represented, so we called Legal Aid to say that there might be situations where we're [working] on a very last-minute basis, so could they set something up so we can move forward as quickly as possible?"

In Ontario the hearing has to take place in front of a judge. Speakman's experience was that judges were very concerned about patient rights, but they were aware of the possible difficulties that preserving those rights might present.

"The other thing the judges were very concerned about was that on the one hand they wanted the person to have the opportunity to be heard, but they didn't want them to be in their courtroom because of the concern of transmission. So we set up electronic transmission of the evidence so the individual would be in a boardroom, for example, and the judge would hear the case but not in the same room.

"It turned out that in Toronto we didn't need to do that. The judges were great. They said, 'You can call us 24 hours a day, seven days a week. 24/7.' No hesitation. 'It has to be done. We'll be available, [there's] a roster, this is who you call.' We had home numbers."

Another issue: serving the order. Under Section 22, compulsory quarantine orders have to be served personally. They could be served by mail, but legally TPH would have to wait seven days for a response, which was out of the question. "We had a really hard time getting process servers. They didn't want to do it. Finally we found somebody in Pickering, which is about twenty miles from here, who was quite willing to get the extra money in his pocket. Public Health made sure he was adequately protected when he was going out. But trying to get those first couple of orders served was difficult."

SARS also brought up new ethical issues, especially concerning rights of privacy. When TPH revealed the name of the son of the index case, "It was not a decision that was made lightly, and it was made in consultation with the family and with their consent. We were very concerned that everybody who might have been in contact with that individual, either at Scarborough Grace or at his mother's funeral-we wanted to make sure that we could reach them."

SARS involved such an urgent need to reach such a large number of unidentified people, the only way to do it was to make broadcast appeals through the mass media—which might have been more efficient than having contact tracers make countless calls, but immediately carried all kinds of risks of breach of privacy.

On another occasion, a nurse who was a SARS suspect rode a commuter train to work and TPH wanted to contact those who had sat near her, but in this case they decided not to release either her name or her photo. "We said, `Hold on a sec. We knew exactly the train she had taken, we knew exactly where she was sitting—we didn't need to release the name." TPH had good descriptions of the six who were sitting by her, but they also followed up with another 26 who insisted that they, too, had sat next to her. "We followed up with 32 of the six people sitting around her," Henry laughed.

* * *

The great social dangers in an epidemic are panic and loss of confidence in authority, both of which drive people to behave in unpredictable ways, ways that may also be reckless and irresponsible, and may help to spread the disease.

Mark Bartlett found himself doing a lot of community education, running around to condominium corporations, doing on-the-fly in-service trainings in businesses.

"There was one I did, I can't say the name but it was a large international beverage manufacturer. They were utterly terrified because one of their staff members had some connections with a case, and they were petrified that their beverage was going to get linked. So I went to their boardroom and gave them an overview that was teleconferenced across the world!"

TPH put out fact sheets and web information in fourteen languages, sending materials to seniors' residences, homeless shelters, church groups, conference planners, provincial jails, doctors' offices, and recreation centers. More than 20,000 handwashing notices alone were sent out to schools and businesses.

Barbara Switzer, a mental health nurse, found herself working almost on her own. The entire mental health team for the city consisted of only eight people, and the manager had just retired so they were somewhat rudderless. She offered psychosocial support to condominium corporations, health care workers in isolation, colleges, schools, community centers, Chinese ESL students, funeral homes, drugstore employees, religious groups, and Canada Post, which was anxious about both quarantine issues and racial profiling.

Her services were also needed at 277 Victoria, where staff were bearing a large portion of the emotional brunt of the outbreak.

A mental health nurse was assigned to each floor, in part to offer help and comfort over the phone to the public, in part to be available to TPH staff who were dealing with confused, angry, grieving, or desperate members of the community. It was especially hard for public health nurses, who are accustomed to being informed and useful, when they didn't have answers, and in some cases could do nothing to help. Switzer wished she had been able to offer group debriefings, but at the end of the day staff just wanted to go home, and at the end of the outbreak the remedy of choice was a long-delayed summer holiday. Several managers said privately that they felt the place suffered from collective post-traumatic stress.

"I don't remember ever driving home during that period," said Anna Miranda, a communicable disease control manager. She calculated that after four weeks of the outbreak she had already worked a month and a half of overtime. "At the end of SARS, just going into the underground parking lot, the smell of it, reminded me of SARS. Even on the eighth floor, there were many of us, myself included, [for whom] it took the longest time to be able to come back up here. It was a whirlwind; it was relentless. It never ended."

* * *

By the end of the outbreak, 700 of TPH's 1,700 employees had worked on SARS.

As a result, everybody in Toronto had suffered, even if they had no contact with SARS. Quit-smoking clinics, various school immunization programs, prenatal counseling sessions, and parenting education groups were all canceled; food safety checks and phone calls and home visits to new mothers were cut back; heart health programming was suspended.

To give one example: while Karietha Cooke was seconded to work on SARS, her own Family Health program was suffering from the loss of personnel, and at the same time needed extra bodies to deal with issues raised by the outbreak. In the one week between the apparent end of the first phase of the outbreak and the apparent beginning of the second, Cooke had to visit a new mother who had just been discharged from a level-three ward. She had to make a home visit, carrying her full protective gear in a bag so the neighbors wouldn't see it, and work out how to be fully masked and gowned before entering the house.

It was during this period of working out in the community that Bonnie Henry realized there was a sad difference between the way that business and public health operated.

At first, a number of businesses refused to let SARS contacts go home and quarantine themselves—who would do their jobs? It took Henry to talk with them about the danger of an infected workplace, and businesses began to see the benefits of quarantine.

TPH also began to see the benefits of backup systems, of disaster planning, and of built-in redundancy. One of the ironies of the situation, in fact, was that no bank thinks of itself as a 21st century institution unless it has an exact replica of its data and its computing system in cases of trouble—yet such a redundancy in a public health care system is characterized as waste.

"We really saw the effects of that when we were desperate for people," Henry said. "Police and fire do a lot better than public health. This was our biggest problem with SARS: we were one deep."

Chapter 13.

Amoy Gardens

The first significant clinical victory against the SARS virus took place on March 29, 2003, when the first batch of Hong Kong SARS patients—medical students and health staff (medical and nursing)—was discharged from the Prince of Wales Hospital. This was a pivotal moment: the outbreak had been growing in Hong Kong for over a month, and these people were the first evidence that one could contract SARS and recover.

Even as they were leaving, though, news was coming in from elsewhere in Kowloon that was very, very disturbing. On March 26, United Christian Hospital called the Kowloon office of the Department of Health to report something strange. Fifteen suspected SARS cases had been admitted in rapid succession. They all came from seven households, and all seven households lived in a housing development called Amoy Gardens.

If Hong Kong is one of the most densely populated regions of the world, Amoy Gardens in turn is one of the most densely populated areas of Hong Kong. The scenic-sounding Amoy Gardens is actually a thicket of 19 needle-thin apartment blocks, a Hong Kong specialty, built in 1981. Each building is 33 floors high, with eight units on each floor, and is home to about a thousand people. If just the complex Amoy Gardens, the size of a few soccer fields, were moved to the state of Vermont in the United States, it would be the second most populous city in the state.

The same day, a team from the Department of Health visited Amoy Gardens, and was puzzled to discover that the affected families lived on seven different floors, didn't know each other and didn't take part in any common activities. They left literature about SARS stressing the importance of hygiene, but were baffled.

Over the next three days, police and experts in water services, environmental protection, electrical and mechanical services, food, environmental hygiene, and drainage all visited Amoy Gardens and came away baffled. Meanwhile, people continued to fall sick at an accelerating rate. By March 30, 190 suspected or confirmed SARS cases had been found from Amoy Gardens, and whole families began fleeing the development.

At dawn on March 31, police wearing surgical masks, gloves, and cloaks cordoned off Block E of Amoy Gardens, and placed all those inside under quarantine. According to the Economist, though, "only 241 tenants in 108 flats were left. The residents of the other 156 flats had already fled—to relations, hotels or friends—possibly spreading the virus they were suspected of carrying with them into the community."

* * *

The Amoy Gardens outbreak was one of the most frightening developments of the SARS outbreak. In every country, so far the majority of the infections had taken place in clusters, and the outbreaks were generally centered on hospitals. The profile of the virus, like the psychological profile of a serial killer, and the efforts to respond to it, had been based on this behavior: this tight, local spread.

Amoy Gardens was different, however: a community outbreak, not just one family or even several people on the same floor of a building, but 329 people in a matter of days. How was the virus spreading? Through air conditioning ducts? Water pipes? Contaminated surfaces such as elevator buttons?

At the time, none of these questions had answers, and suddenly it seemed as if no one was safe. The effect of the Amoy Gardens outbreak was to raise the level of alarm in Hong Kong to the highest levels. Professor Jen-Fu Chiu, who had recently moved to Hong Kong after teaching for more than 20 years in the United States, said, "It was like being at war."

Schools and universities closed. Restaurants emptied. Supermarkets were full, as people stocked up with provisions, especially after an unfounded rumor began circulating that the whole of Hong Kong might be quarantined. Rush hour dissipated, as people tried to avoid contact by working at home or taking public transport at off-peak hours. Some used their own cars, normally a high-overhead option in Hong Kong. On a bus or the MTR subway, everyone wore masks. Anyone not wearing a mask would get dark looks, because there was an implied selfishness: the mask protected others from you, as well as you from others.

Some, like Ella To, recently retired after a lifetime of teaching, left the province around April 1, disturbed by seeing masks even in the supermarkets, and stayed with her sons in Australia.

HSBC, the city's main bank, closed a floor of its main office after an employee showed symptoms, and sent 50 traders home for a week as a precaution. PCCW (Hong Kong's dominant telecom provider), Hewlett-Packard, and Intel sent their staff home. Tourism virtually came to a screeching halt: hotels were mostly empty; concerts were canceled. Inbound business travel slowed to a trickle, and the Hong Kong stock market fell to a four-and-a-half-year low. A reporter for the Economist wrote: "Whenever people do meet-masked, invariably—a surreal mixture of anxiety and denial hangs in the air."

In some respects, Hong Kong pioneered public infection-control tactics, the street scenes, and what might be called the SARS way of life.

People wore masks almost everywhere in public: in stores, on trains and buses, in offices. Someone making his way around the province might be temperature-tested as many as a dozen times a day—going into shopping centers, getting onto ferries, at border crossings, railway stations, at the entrances to hospitals and Ministry of Health buildings, in some places with the digital thermometer in the ear, in others with the infrared cameras that read the heat coming off the body and warned if it was over 37°C.

Buses were disinfected constantly: a daily scrubdown inside and out with disinfectant—especially the tires—and sprayed periodically during the day again. Anything that multiple people touched with their hands—the belts of escalators in particular—was disinfected almost constantly, and people avoided touching them whenever possible.

Everyone's peace of mind was tormented by rumor. Karen Richardson of the Asian edition of the *Wall Street Journal* was stationed in Hong Kong during the outbreak.

"There were rumors circulating all over the city. The local papers were printing front-page color schematics of possible spreading routes. I saw a kind of three-dimensional color diagram on the front page of one local paper that actually had a drawing of a construction worker urinating off the side of a building while standing up on a bamboo scaffolding. The diagram showed with numbers or arrows how the wind may have blown his urine into an open window, and then spread SARS throughout the building. That rumor got a lot of airtime on radio shows and column inches in newspapers.

"Everyone feared that their building was going to be the next Amoy Gardens. Some people put together a website to identify all the buildings in Hong Kong that had cases in them. You knew it wasn't accurate; it wasn't sponsored by the government, and so eventually the government had to put up its own website with all the buildings. Just to give you a sense of the paranoia, there was a phone service where you could actually dial a number and find out if you were standing within a kilometer of an infected building. We went to talk to these people [running the service] and they had a lot of subscribers."

There was even a kind of SARS spam. "I received several emails, [copied to] tons of people, about various buildings, including the Citibank Tower and the Bank of China building, in the financial district being infected and evacuated. I spent several hours trying to verify them. It turned out some of these rumors were possibly started by competitors."

University classes resumed before public schools went back. Even so, Mary Waye said, everyone at the Chinese University still had to wear masks indoors for a couple of weeks. She even had to lecture in a mask. "I have quite a soft voice. People can barely hear me without a mask!"

Meanwhile, Professor Waye had two children home from school, with all the conventional children's activities outside the home suspended. For some parents, she said, it was an opportunity to stay home with their children, but that was not an option for her. Her nine-year-old daughter Jade was lucky enough to have a close friend, Bo-Bo, whose mother was trusting enough to invite her over to play, but even then, Waye said, "You have to tell your little girl how to use the elevator: 'If you touch the button, don't touch your face.'" Her seven-year-old son Fred was sometimes looked after by a maid, sometimes by a neighbor. One night, coming home exhausted, she was greeted by her daughter with tears in her eyes demanding to know why her mommy couldn't take a few days off and take care of her just like the other mommies.

When the schools reopened, parents had to fill out and sign a form before a child would be allowed to go to school, saying that they had taken their child's temperature, and giving the reading. Even so, the children would line up to be let into school, and their temperatures were taken (in the ear or on the forehead, depending on the equipment) every time they entered the building. Recess time was extended to allow time for the children to wash their hands in extra makeshift sinks that were built for the occasion in the playground.

It was a very tense time. One day Waye's husband came home and told her he'd just found out that the friend of a technician who had come in to work on the air conditioner in the office had come down with SARS. Her husband wasn't sure how much risk was involved—but he had also started to develop a sore throat. What should they do? In the end, they decided that to be on the safe side he should go into voluntary home quarantine, and the rest of the family would stay clear of him.

The media attention was an added strain. Waye, like many scientists involved in SARS work, faced constant requests from reporters, many of which involved a delicate disentangling of fact and fiction, or were beyond their knowledge. Was it sound to treat SARS patients with high doses of steroids? Sometimes the questions could take a long time to explain or were just too off-topic to consider: Waye received a letter from someone who asked if SARS was caused by consuming too much genetically engineered food. Meanwhile, there remained an urgent need to sequence more strains of SARS that might have different virulence patterns—such as giving diarrhea in addition to the respiratory symptoms—work which stretched the limit of the already strained team.

Above all, it was a landscape of uncertainty.

"Every time you had a bit of a fever or you felt as if you might have a bit of a fever," said Dr. Paul Tam, Chief of Pediatric Surgery at the University of Hong Kong, "you wondered. I was in a meeting and someone turned off the air conditioning and I felt a bit sweaty, and I wondered. And being a doctor, you always think about the worst outcome. And the worst outcome did happen." One of his colleagues, Dr James Lau, who was his senior at Queen Mary Hospital, was the first doctor to die of SARS. "It makes you feel vulnerable. It can happen. It can happen to people around you. We started going to funerals and memorial services. . . ." He paused, looking down. "The university has lost several of its graduates, several young doctors, too. It touches the heart." He broke off.

* * *

Amoy Gardens remained on the fringes of everyone's awareness, like a haunted house on the edge of town. Over the next few weeks, intensive investigation turned up a likely, though not definitive chain of events. First, a patient was sent home from hospital too soon, and once the patient was back in Amoy Gardens, another unexpected feature of the virus came into play: during the infectious phase of the illness, a patient sheds large quantities of live virus not only by coughing and sneezing, but also in feces. This might have had no ill effect but for the first of several coincidental factors: the Amoy Gardens sewage outflow pipe suffered some kind of blockage and sewage began to leak and back up.

Again, this might not have been especially dangerous were it not for two other factors. In many of the apartments, the U-bends or water traps had dried up, and sewer gases rose up the outflow pipes and back into the apartments. At the same time, the particular configuration of the buildings combined with the wind flow at the time to create a "wind curtain" effect, cutting off the draft through the complex and setting up a stagnant well of air between the buildings that allowed the airborne virus to rise slowly and seep in through the open apartment windows. It's possible that yet another factor involved exhaust fans: as the foul-smelling sewer gases entered the apartment bathrooms, those residents who had exhaust fans in their bathrooms turned them on and shut the bathroom doors—thereby creating a negative air pressure that sucked more infected air up from the sewer.

Were other factors at play too? As late as August, it was proposed that SARS had been spread by infected rats—a familiar enemy from the days of plague.

The Food and Environmental Hygiene Department set 100 mousetraps a day for about two months but caught only 14 rats, which suggests that infestation was mild. The Amoy Gardens outbreak peaked in just a few days, and it seemed unlikely that rats could spread the disease over so many apartments so rapidly unless there were a considerable number of infected rats. Moreover, rats in Hong Kong fall into two species: rattus norvegicus, the Norwegian or sewer rat, and rattus rattus, the roof rat. The two species are territorial: the sewer rats, as their name suggests, tend to inhabit sewers and underground regions; the roof rats live higher up. Given the location of the infections, the culprits would have to be roof rats. Of the 14 rats trapped in the infected Amoy Gardens apartments, only one was a roof rat, and it showed no sign of SARS infection. Although some of the remaining 13 sewer rats showed traces of SARS coronavirus, it was not in their blood; the rats were not infected. They had likely picked up some virus in the sewers, but they had almost certainly not passed it on to the residents of the Amoy Gardens apartments.

Other suspects such as cockroaches were investigated by Dr. Thomas Tsang of the Ministry of Health, who had also investigated the Metropole. "We say that rodents and cockroaches have a part to play as mechanical carriers because we found samples of coronavirus genetic material on the cockroaches and also rodent droppings. We believe that they could have been carrying contaminated feces, especially from the sewage drains and from one place to another, thus contributing to the spread of infection. Now, luckily, we only found them in the droppings and also the service swabs. There is no evidence that they are actually replicating in the carriers—the rats and the cockroaches themselves. Were this the case, the scale of the outbreak would even be much bigger."

But this is all hindsight. The lack of immediate answers to the epidemiological and zoonotic investigations at both the Metropole and Amoy Gardens had a withering effect everywhere in the world. For the next three months, nobody could be sure that the virus was really spread only in droplet form, and only by close contact. (To this day people in Hong Kong are still wary of elevator buttons.) Though the gathering evidence and the rational mind said that this was almost always the case, even in the most qualified and phlegmatic minds of public health there was a persistent unease that, under the wrong circumstances, the virus would break out into the community, cases would turn up at the hospitals in the hundreds each day, contact tracing would be overwhelmed, containment would be impossible, and everything would collapse.

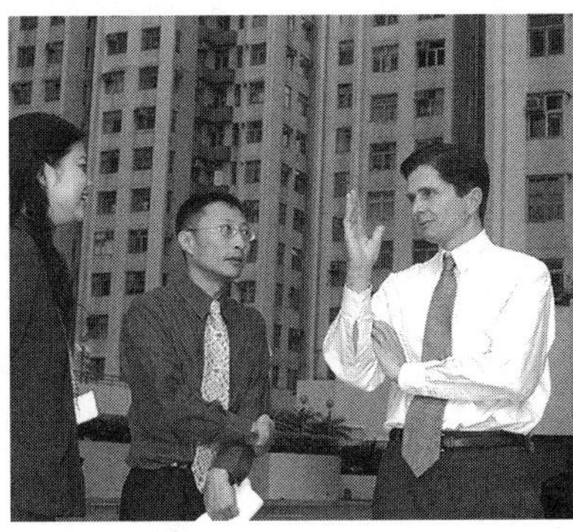

The World Health Organization's Executive Director for Communicable Diseases, Dr. David L. Heymann, right, visiting the Amoy Gardens housing estate in Ngau Tau Kok, where one block had to be evacuated.

Photograph courtesy of Information Services Department of the Hong Kong SAR Government

Chapter 14.

Removing the Handle

In 1853, London suffered one of its periodic outbreaks of cholera, a water-borne infectious disease still common in parts of the world. John Snow, a London physician, was curious that deaths from this severe, debilitating diarrhea seemed to occur in a cluster. He began mapping the cases and interviewing the surviving patients and their families, wondering what they had in common, asking about what they had consumed, where they had been recently, and what they had done.

Snow discovered that they all took their water from a water pump on Broad Street in central London. He didn't know what the exact link between the cholera and the pump was—the organism that causes cholera (*Vibrio cholerae*) wasn't discovered for another 30 years—but the water from that pump clearly had something to do with the outbreak. In what was probably the first and certainly the cheapest intervention in the history of epidemiology, he asked to have the pump handle removed. People grumbled and had to fetch their water from other sources farther away, but the outbreak stopped.

With SARS, the "handle" was international air travel. If the case of the Singaporean doctor pulled off the plane in Frankfurt hadn't been enough to convince the WHO that people with SARS would carry the virus around the world even after the global advisory, two more cases over the next few days—also involving physicians—would have been persuasive on their own.

The international character of the French Hospital in Hanoi meant that it was a potential port of arrival for an international traveler with SARS; and because it was staffed largely by French doctors on brief rotations, the hospital also provided a point of international departure for SARS.

One of the doctors, on an Air France flight home, infected two others on the flight, unwittingly giving researchers valuable information about how SARS might be transmitted within a plane.

We'll call him Dr. A. On March 22, 2003, he boarded the Air France Hanoi-Bangkok-Paris flight of March 22-23. The flight had 30 flight crew and 371 passengers: 166 boarded in Hanoi, and at Bangkok 5 left the plane and 205 others boarded.

Dr. A was already infected before he got on the plane and sat in seat 26L. Seven people sat within two rows of his seat; two said they had noticed that he was pale and breathing rapidly through pursed lips during the flight. He left his seat at least twice between Bangkok and Paris to go to the front lavatory. During the stopover in Bangkok, he got off with the passengers leaving and then got back on before the passengers who embarked in Bangkok. When the plane landed in Paris, he was cared for by the airport medical services, along with two other physicians who had worked in the French Hospital in Hanoi and were on the same plane.

Of the seven passengers who sat within two rows of him, SARS developed in only Patient B, sitting in seat 25K, who handled the same aircraft magazines and used the same lavatory as Dr. A. (Owing to the layout of the plane, Dr. A also passed next to seat 25K on the way to the lavatory.) Another passenger who sat nearby, in seat 26K, reported a sore throat and a temperature of 37.6°C once during follow-up, but nothing else.

In this case, the WHO guidelines for screening aircraft passengers fitted real-world experience only up to a point. The guidelines assumed the passengers sitting within two rows of an infected person were at greatest risk, and should be quarantined at home for 10 days after exposure and contacted daily by telephone. Patient C, though, was something of a mystery. He boarded the plane in Bangkok, sat in seat 30B, didn't know Dr. A and had nothing to do with him during the flight. He used the toilets at the rear, rather than the front, and was one of the first to leave the plane. (On a Hong Kong-Beijing flight at almost exactly the same time, a passenger with SARS in row 14 seems to have infected three patients in row 12 and one in row 9.)

Of Dr. A's other contacts, two people who shared the same car to the Hanoi airport, two taxi drivers, four health care workers who had treated him at Paris Charles de Gaulle Airport, and the two doctors who left the plane with him, none showed any signs of SARS. This was despite their having been in much closer proximity to Dr. A than the other passengers on the plane. The virus was as capricious as ever.

Another doctor from the French Hospital was intercepted just in time. "Doctors were working for two to three weeks," WHO's Pascale Brudon recounted, "so we knew that a number of doctors who had been [working] at the hospital were leaving the country. We discussed this with the French Hospital and told them they needed to check [the doctors], and only those they felt were okay should be allowed to leave. And we rechecked them ourselves; either by telephone, or one of my staff would visit them and interview them. But one of them, a doctor who died later here in Viet Nam, was not approved by the hospital. He was apparently not very well, and they said he should wait for a while before going home—and we couldn't interview him because he was not staying at the same hotel."

Knowing that a number of people were planning to leave, Brudon wisely provided all the airlines with a check sheet for passengers, warning them about the danger signs. "Everyone was so afraid at that time that they were all aware of what to look for. The guy at the airline desk knew what was going on, and he called me and asked if we had interviewed all the doctors leaving the country. I said, 'No.' Then he called the French Hospital and [the doctor] was not allowed on the plane."

This act of quarantine may have protected the passengers and crew of the plane, and everyone at the plane's destination, but it had its drawbacks: the doctor went back to stay with his friends, who unfortunately contracted SARS from him.

At that point, Brudon added, the WHO had put out the global travel alert but the International Air Transport Association (IATA) had not yet given any instructions to the airlines. "So the airlines were very reluctant to give out any information in the plane, or to [warn] the passengers, 'If you feel ill, go to your doctor.' So we did it [instead], and some of the airlines agreed to distribute it to their staff and to passengers."

* * *

Between March 15 and 20, cases were suspected in Indonesia, United Kingdom, Australia, Bahrain, the Philippines, Israel, Germany, Brunei, Thailand, Ireland, Japan, France, Spain, Switzerland, Malaysia, and Finland. Heymann knew the WHO had to act.

"With all this in mind," he said later, "we knew we had to do something more serious. We made a determined decision that we would do two things: we would start a global containment action to try to prevent this disease from becoming a pandemic, and at the same time we would try to get real-time information from collaborators. So that's what we did. Between the 15th and the 27th we got information that people were traveling internationally with the disease; that an unknown number of people were getting sick on airplanes that were carrying those people. In fact someone we all knew from here [another international organization based in Geneva] was traveling between Thailand and Beijing, and got sick and died. We had a staff member, Dr. Urbani, who had got sick and died. We also knew that some businessmen had gone back to Taiwan from Hong Kong and had got sick when they got home. We knew that this was serious.

"So with this information, we made a recommendation on the 27th of March about two things: one, if a person was a contact, they shouldn't travel; and two, if the person was sick with symptoms that looked like SARS, they shouldn't travel."

At this point, there were still no bans, advisories, or embargoes against specific countries or areas. However, by now the WHO was entering two other sets of turf: other countries' and the airlines'.

"We talked with IATA, we talked with representatives of the airline industry before we made these recommendations, and they agreed with them. Then we put the recommendations out and let the [individual] countries decide how they would operationalize them. This was for every country with outbreaks: you make you own decision on how you want to operationalize them."

Heymann was trying to make a fine distinction between being the world's doctor and the world's policeman. "We said, 'Ask two questions. Have you had contact? Are you sick?'"

How individual countries implemented these recommendations varied enormously. "Hong Kong had stop points at their immigration where they had the contact lists. When you came in through immigration they looked first to see if your name was on the contact list. Their system was incredibly intricate. If your name was on the stop list, you didn't go through. If you got through there you had to fill out a health declaration saying you weren't sick, and then they checked you. But Canada had a booth that you walked by on your way to register for the flight, and you could pick [a flier] up if you wanted to; it asked you two questions. It was a passive system."

Not only was the implementation of the screening process enacted in varying ways, but by now countries were beginning to issue their own advisories. On March 19, Health Canada suggested people should postpone travel to high-risk parts of Southeast Asia, including Viet Nam and Singapore. This was advice that would later come back to haunt them. Canada issued an advisory that covered the whole of Viet Nam even though the outbreak was limited to one hospital in Hanoi; later, Canadians would howl in protest when the WHO issued an advisory for Toronto even though the outbreak was limited to hospitals.

"One of the reasons we decided to go ahead and make our own travel recommendations," Heymann said, "was that countries were making their own recommendations based on no evidence. The United States and Canada and the United Kingdom all had travel advisories that were confusing everybody. Without any evidence."

The crucial factor, though, was Amoy Gardens. The epidemiological mystery in Kowloon would have repercussions around the world. It was still early in the outbreak—the disease had been named less than two weeks previously—and this large, sudden, unexplained community spread scared everyone. Before Amoy Gardens, it had been assumed that you were probably safe if you avoided close contact with other people with SARS. For several weeks after Amoy Gardens, all bets were off. The WHO, Heymann explained, could no longer safely say, "Yes, you can go to Hong Kong as long as you avoid people with SARS." There was the nagging possibility that if you were in an outbreak area you might catch SARS by some unknown means, without close personal contact.

"Between the 27th of March and the 2nd of April we got more information: something was transmitting this in the environment, in Hong Kong. At the same time we became aware that whereas previously contact tracing was linked in every case to a previous case, we now had some cases that couldn't be linked to a previous case. Was this because there was an environmental factor? Was this because there were asymptomatic people who were transmitting the disease?" This was the Typhoid Mary fear—that someone who is apparently quite healthy passes the disease on to scores of others.

"We didn't know, but we made the decision that we needed to be more severe in the case of countries where outbreaks of significance were occurring, so people didn't go there and get infection from a source that was not yet understood."

The WHO began to make travel recommendations based on several criteria, including the size of the epidemic, and whether or not they could trace all of their cases to another case. On April 2, after carefully explaining its data and reasoning, the organization issued this travel advice:

"As a measure of precaution WHO is now recommending that persons traveling to Hong Kong and Guangdong Province of China consider postponing all but essential travel. This temporary recommendation will be reassessed in the light of the evolution of the epidemic in the areas currently indicated, and other areas of the world could become subject to similar recommendations if the situation demands. Please note that this recommendation applies only to travelers entering Hong Kong Special Administrative Region of China and Guangdong Province of China, not to passengers directly transiting through international airports within those areas."

The WHO advice was precautionary, rather than a travel ban. Individual governments, however, were not as restrained. Over the next few days, for example, the U.S. State Department authorized all nonessential employees and their families to leave the province of Guangdong. Malaysia and Japan issued travel advisories warning their citizens not to travel to Canada. On May 15 2003, Australia and New Zealand issued new travel alerts for several countries in Southeast Asia, advising travelers to be especially careful in countries such as Singapore, Malaysia, and Thailand, even though Malaysia and Thailand suffered outbreaks that were minor at worst. The Vietnamese government forbade Vietnamese nationals to travel to Taiwan for work. New Zealand turned a Chinese delegation of 43 away from a conference but this had not quite the irony of Italy barring people from China, Hong Kong, and Taiwan from the Far East Film Festival, an annual showcase of Asian films. Meanwhile, traders from China, Hong Kong, Singapore, and Viet Nam were barred from one of the world's biggest jewelry and watch fairs in Switzerland.

Various countries in Asia tightened rules on people entering, as well as on certain behaviors. Two days after Malaysia stopped almost all holders of Hong Kong and China passports from entering the country, China banned organized tours to Malaysia, Singapore, and Thailand. Indonesia warned its citizens to stop spitting in public. The Philippines advised against unnecessary travel to either Hong Kong or Guangdong. Roman Catholic priests in Singapore were asked to stop hearing confessions, because of the close proximity of the confessional.

In the words of the Straits Times, "The whole of eastern Asia was being placed in involuntary quarantine."

* * *

The general results of this "quarantine" are now well known, though the details are still startling.

By mid-April, Thailand, although a non-SARS country, had seen 50,000 cancellations at hotels for April and May, mostly by Western tourists. In mid-May, the Economist reported that Hong Kong's hotel occupancy rate was at an abnormally low 15 percent instead of the usual 82 percent, and Singapore's tourism was down by 67 percent. Economic projections from the World Travel & Tourism Council pegged Viet Nam to lose 15 percent of its 2003 tourism industry income, with Singapore and Hong King losing almost triple that percentage at 43 percent and 41 percent, respectively.

On a single day, one-third of all flights in and out of Hong Kong airport were canceled. Singapore International Airlines (SIA) canceled all flights to Guangzhou, Cathay Pacific canceled Malaysia altogether, and Taiwan was said to consider suspending air links to China. ANA, a Japanese airline, reported that passenger traffic between Tokyo and Hong Kong fell by one-fifth after the disease was identified. Qantas cut 20 percent of its total international flights: this, with SARS still affecting a relatively small geographic area. Even Disney warned investors that SARS would have a noticeable impact on its profits because fewer people were flying to America to visit its theme parks.

Of all the suffering airlines, Hong Kong-based Cathay Pacific was probably hit hardest. Even before the first travel advisories, it met with the worst publicity possible when a headline in The Standard of March 21 read: "VIRUS MAN FLEW CATHAY." It continued, "A man on a Cathay Pacific flight to London from Hong Kong has possibly become the third Briton to contract the killer pneumonia." In mid-April, a leaked internal memo said that passenger numbers had fallen from 30,000 daily to 10,000; if they fell as far as 6,000 a day, the airline might have to ground its entire fleet. On May 10, the Economist reported that Cathay was asking staff to take unpaid leave as passenger numbers were 75 percent down from a year previously.

Cathay chief executive David Turnbull said a combination of SARS and the Iraq war "has annihilated our passenger bookings."

The calculus of disaster is never exact, but the WHO announced, "Preliminary estimates have placed the cost of the outbreak at nearly US$100 billion, mainly as a result of canceled travel and decreased investment in Asia alone."

* * *

It wasn't just eastern Asia that was being placed in involuntary quarantine. Few actions anywhere in the world caused such outcry as the WHO travel advisories concerning Canada.

On April 23, 2003, having issued SARS updates more or less daily but having left its travel recommendations unchanged for three weeks, the WHO announced:

"As a result of ongoing assessments as to the nature of outbreaks of severe acute respiratory syndrome (SARS) in Beijing and Shanxi Province, China, and in Toronto, Canada, WHO is now recommending, as a measure of precaution, that persons planning to travel to these destinations consider postponing all but essential travel."

Toronto's mayor was almost incoherent with fury. Sheela Basrur, the medical officer of health said that to link Toronto with China was a "gross misrepresentation of the facts" because the disease was not spreading through the community. Health Canada sent a formal letter of protest to the WHO demanding that it take back its Toronto travel advisory, claiming that the WHO based its warning on outdated information. Other parties weighed in: the CDC in Atlanta said that a travel advisory for Toronto was unwarranted, but British medical officers supported the advisory.

As if this first phase were not contentious enough, six days later the WHO lifted the advisory, yet a little over three weeks later it became clear that SARS was by no means finished with Ontario, and a second phase of the outbreak began.

The rights and wrongs of the situation will probably never be resolved. It's quite possible the WHO was working from less than current data, given the circumstances recounted in Chapter 12. On the other hand, the protests on April 29 when the advisory was lifted suggest that Torontonians felt there was something whimsical about the advisories, which seems very unlikely.

From an outsider's point of view, two observations seem worth making. First, the WHO, like its parent, the United Nations, is in a curious position on the world pecking order of nations. While some nations seem to see the world body as large and important, capable of bringing in expertise, information, and equipment they lack, others clearly like to see themselves as being above such necessity. Some First World countries would never call in the WHO out of need; others would never call in the WHO out of principle. It's hard to say where Canada fits in this hierarchy, but it seems clear that while Canadians had no problem with the WHO issuing advisories for Asian nations, it was quite a different matter to issue an advisory for a major North American city.

Second, in listening to members of Toronto Public Health talk about the travel advisory, and in a broader sense hearing them describe what the WHO did and didn't do for the city, one comes away with the impression that the outrage at the advisory was a focal point for a broader sense of grievance. If one can generalize about a complex bureaucracy of 1,700 employees, TPH felt overextended and abandoned by the province, Health Canada, and, in the person of the WHO, the world.

The WHO was seen largely as an irritant, demanding information that TPH had no time to research and provide. In TPH's perception, the organization did little to bring them useful information from elsewhere in the world. One suspects the Canadian exasperation at the travel advisories was perhaps as much an expression of these frustrations as anything else.

Whatever the rights and wrongs, the impact of the announcement was undeniable. The city was twice cursed: not only by the advisory, but by the impression given in the media that Torontonians were dropping like flies on every street corner.

"The perception that travel to Toronto was unsafe," wrote the *New York Times*, "was based on relentless news media coverage as the death count rose to about 40, making the city the most affected outside Asia."

"Perception versus reality was just so skewed," said Rod Seiling, president of the Greater Toronto Hotel Association. In mid-June, a consulting firm reported that the tourism industry in Toronto had lost nearly $190 million because of the SARS outbreak. ""The impact is profound," Lyle Hall, managing director of a hospitality, leisure, and tourism company, said in a release. "We have never seen revenue losses of this magnitude and across all sectors, not only accommodation, but also restaurants, attractions, transportation companies, and tour operators."

Not only did Toronto lose hotel, theater, bus, tour, restaurant, and convention business, but the province of Ontario reckoned that hotel cancellations cost $60 million in April alone, even while the province was facing a health care bill for the outbreak that would rise above $900 million. And the old joke that Americans know nothing about Canadian geography came home to roost: summer camps in not only Ontario but British Columbia and Quebec reported a sharp drop in enrollments from the United States, and parents farther afield were apparently under the impression that all of Canada was stricken with SARS.

Camp Manitou in Muskoka, whose website helpfully provides flight schedules for campers arriving from Paris, Los Angeles, Miami, and New York, had 24 campers from Mexico cancel. "They phoned me up and said they'd heard 2,000 people here died of SARS," said Mark Diamond, the camp's co-owner.

Luc Dubois, president of the 38-year-old Edphy International Camp in Val-Morin, Quebec—a province without a single SARS case—tried to allay parents' fears with newsletters every two days and maps illustrating the distance between Toronto and Montreal relative to distances in the campers' home countries. "People thought Montreal and Toronto were side-by-side," he said. According to him, the one group that seemed to take the SARS scare in stride were Africans—perhaps, he suggested, because Africa is used to virus scares, and Africans recognize that even if one country suffers an outbreak, that doesn't mean the whole continent is unsafe.

* * *

There was a postscript to the vexing issue of travel advisories and bans. Heymann points out that the first WHO advisories were in fact aimed at preventing in-flight infection, and after the March 27 advisory, no cases of SARS seem to have been caused by this means. He also argues that rather than causing panic and stigma, evidence-based travel advice was used by the public as "a benchmark" of the progress of the fight against SARS in those areas. By being neither hysterical nor adversarial, the WHO information could then be used to regain world confidence after an area was declared safe.

As one piece of evidence to support this view, he cites the rapid rebound in passenger figures from Hong Kong airport. The low point—just before May 23, 2003, when the travel recommendations were removed—was 14,670 a day. Then the advisory was lifted, and passenger numbers rose more than 350 percent to 54,195 on July 12, little more than a month later. It did indeed seem the advice was seen as authoritative and trustworthy—even if, as others claimed, it erred on the side of caution.

In late June the *Economist* reported that China, which was in some respects hit the hardest by SARS, was likely to achieve at least 7 percent growth over the year, "only a percentage point or so below what the country would probably have achieved without SARS." Certainly, many other affected countries did not enjoy as robust an economy as China's. Yet for all the dire predictions of a global outbreak of long-term economic catastrophe, the various micro- and macro-economies took a hit, staggered, and survived.

Chapter 15.

Singapore: A Case Study in Quarantine

By mid-March 2003, it looked as though SARS had been contained in Singapore. Then a series of new cases appeared: epidemiological tracking showed that three index cases resulted in 21 primary contacts developing SARS, who in turn infected up to 41 other people.

As a result, on March 24, the government decided to take a step that was criticized by other nations as "draconian," and would certainly have posed civil liberties problems elsewhere on the globe. The Singapore Ministry of Health said that for the first time in 33 years it would be invoking the Infectious Diseases Act to isolate for 10 days everyone who had been exposed to infected SARS patients. Under most circumstances, quarantine would have to take place at home; in some cases, as we'll see, it would be in other settings.

Quarantine was one of the central issues of the outbreak, but it turned out to be a far more difficult and contentious issue than authorities expected. The idea of removing potentially infected people from circulation seemed, frankly, a no-brainer; yet administering and enforcing quarantine turned out to create dozens of downstream problems. The paradox of taking innocent people and treating them almost like criminals was extremely hard to resolve, and in the end it wasn't clear whether quarantine was essential after all. Given that this issue will face every country in the grip of an outbreak of infectious disease—especially an unknown one—it is instructive to take a closer look at the Singapore story.

The government's first step was to convince everyone to take quarantine seriously, or else the exercise would be pointless. The National Environment Agency's head of quarantine and epidemiology, Dr. Goh Kee Tai, announced that breach of quarantine would result in a fine of $5,000 for a first offense, and $10,000 for a second.

Yet while this provision was giving the impression that those under quarantine were potential criminals, it was also clear that they were innocent of any wrongdoing, and to insist that those who were quarantined wouldn't be allowed leave the house even to buy groceries meant that the government was therefore also obliged to find someone else to do the shopping for them. From somewhere an entirely new organization would have to be concocted to help them out in this state of innocent imprisonment—and also to be their jailers, making sure that they were at home as ordered.

Finally, those in quarantine fell into yet a third category: they had been exposed to a potentially lethal virus, and might fall deadly ill (and deadly infectious) at any time. This meant in turn that whatever SARS task force was created, as the Minister promised, would also have to be able to monitor the health of those in quarantine; if anybody developed symptoms of the disease, they would need referral to Tan Tock Seng Hospital or the Communicable Disease Centre (CDC). It was hard to say which were more tangled: the ethical issues involved, or the administrative ones.

Calls started going out to over 700 people: 279 family members of SARS patients, 47 colleagues, 52 friends and acquaintances, plus 140 preschoolers and 200 students from Pei Cai Secondary School whose classmates were suspected of having the virus. They were to stay home, wear a mask in the presence of family members, take their temperature, and report any suspicious symptoms.

Osman David Mansoor, of the Western Pacific (WPRO) branch of the WHO in Manila, said: "What we have seen in Singapore, from the WHO point of view, is appropriate action, given that you have to balance control and allow people to do things without totally inhibiting their movement. Singapore has taken even more precautions than the WHO has recommended. You're ultra-cautious. That's obviously a very good thing."

Not everyone agreed. A number of voices from other countries voiced the opinion that Singapore was behaving like a police state—though these opinions tended to originate from countries that had few or no SARS cases.

At once, the numbers started to rise. By the end of the day, about 600 to 700 school children had been sent home. The following day, the government decided to close all primary schools, secondary schools, junior colleges, and centralized institutes until April 6, 2003, later amended to April 7. Some 600,000 children were told to stay home.

In a joint statement issued in Singapore on March 24, the Ministries of Education and Health said, "On purely medical grounds, there are currently no strong reasons for closing all schools. However, principals and general practitioners have reported that parents continue to be concerned about the risk to their children in schools."

It was a paradoxical situation: the government appeared to be acting in a fashion some thought was authoritarian, yet it was pressure from parents, and perhaps anxiety on the part of the school authorities, that had brought about the school closures. (Almost identical issues would arise in Toronto.) In a sense, as an editorial in the Straits Times observed, the public was imposing home quarantine on itself.

All school competitions and extracurricular activities were canceled or postponed. Preschool centers also closed, as did child care facilities, playgroups, special education schools, tuition classes at community centers/clubs, and residents' committees and madrasahs (Islamic religious schools). The last time Singapore schools had been closed on such a massive scale was in 1958, when 250,000 students stayed home during a particularly virulent polio outbreak.

This time, only the universities, polytechnics, and institutes of technical education were unaffected, as they had older students who "are better able to understand the situation and take the necessary precautions," said Rear-Admiral Teo Chee Hean, the Education Minister. Confident words—but almost at once the government closed the Ngee Ann Polytechnic for a week after a student contracted SARS from his mother, who had died from the disease.

Closing the schools, like many aspects of quarantine, solved one problem but caused another. "When we close the schools tomorrow," urged Lim Hng Kiang, the Health Minister, "I hope parents don't take it lightly and send all their kids to the shopping centers and they congregate there. Then it defeats the whole purpose."

He was right to be wary: once the schools closed, the children of Singapore presented a vast logistical problem to their parents—especially parents who themselves were quarantined, and thus severely handicapped in their ability to cope with their children.

In a sense the problem faced by the whole of Singapore had been broken down into small pieces and handed out to unprepared individuals and families. At once, this created a sort of Hydra, with 3.3 million heads, each in turn a potential problem for the authorities and the population in general. The children were the first demonstration of the difficulties of quarantine: some went to the malls, some went to the cinemas, and about 175 even visited countries where SARS was rampant.

* * *

These difficulties were a tip-off that voluntary quarantine was implicitly based on the "quarantinee" being a responsible, autonomous adult with a stable living situation. Children didn't fit into that category. People who spoke nonmainstream languages presented problems everywhere, as did the elderly, the anxious, and the easily confused. Special difficulties also arose dealing with various other sub-populations: the homeless, inmates in jails, and the elderly and dependent who needed care in nursing homes.

Toronto Public Health realized early that all three raised major problems on two fronts: all were extremely difficult to isolate and sustain, and they could be dangerously fertile ground for the virus. "If SARS got into that population," said Bonnie Henry, speaking of the homeless in Toronto, "it would be devastating. How do you quarantine someone who's in a shelter?"

Similarly, Toronto's two large jails, one of which had already been described by a judge as "medieval," were extremely vulnerable. Jails would seem to exist already as a form of quarantine, but here, too, things didn't quite go as planned. At first, the jails tried screening all incoming inmates, asking about fevers and contacts, but the men caught on quickly and began saying, Oh yes, definitely, lots of contacts. "That way," Bonnie Henry explained dryly, "instead of being sent to the cells they'd go to hospital and talk to a nice nurse."

The jails also decided to stop all visitors, to prevent the virus being brought in or out, but that backfired, too. "The downstream effect of that was that inmates in the jail were so lonely that they would call our hotline at eleven o'clock at night so they could talk to a nurse! And to complain, of course, about not having visitors."

And what about people who lived in social structures different from the usual semi-detached family life? In Toronto, explained Bonnie Henry, "there was a very close-knit religious community where people were quarantined over the Easter weekend, which was an important holiday for them, and people were concerned about missing the church service. So we helped them with arrangements to have the church service by cable television, and door-to-door delivery of the host. Those are the sorts of things that allow you to suffer through a ...not very pleasant situation."

* * *

One of the most difficult issues that Singapore, like other nations, faced was the question of how much quarantine was necessary. Even to have the 10-day rule of thumb, suggested by the WHO, must have been a thin but vital straw: indefinite quarantine must have seemed like a life sentence. Nobody knew who would be affected, who would be most affected, how much to worry, and how far to go in trying to set up alternative arrangements.

Equally, nobody knew exactly what the experience of being quarantined would be like, or how the public would react to it. At first, it mostly seemed surprisingly banal, a matter of domestic arrangements. Four-year-old Joseph Teo was quarantined along with the other students at his preschool, where a five-year-old was diagnosed with SARS. The Ministry of Health delivered a quarantine letter which stated he was to stay home for 10 days, minimize contact with family and friends, cover his mouth and nose when he coughed or sneezed, and to take his temperature every day. His seven-year-old sister Jolene was also told to stay home with similar instructions.

"It's a good thing I have my maid at home to help look after both of them," their mother said. A good thing for Mrs. Teo, that is; in the coming days one maid would catch SARS from her employer and 19 others would be quarantined along with their employing families.

The sense of isolation would turn out to be one of the greatest hardships of the quarantine, and one of the greatest incentives to break it. By May, volunteers from a neighborhood SARS task force were lending their personal cellular phones to quarantined people who had no telephone at home.

* * *

Meanwhile, events were taking place that would make the simple edict of quarantine even more complicated. Two days after the quarantine law had been put into effect, early in the morning of Wednesday, March 26, a Singapore woman we'll call Tsui Mei-ling flew into Changi airport on China Southern Airlines flight CZ 355.

A marketing manager of a company which designs, plans, and manages conferences, exhibitions, and other corporate events, Tsui had left Singapore on March 14, the day the government started advising people against traveling to SARS-hit areas. She was in Hong Kong for two days before going to Beijing, where she developed a fever on March 19. She saw one hospital doctor who put her on a drip for a few hours and then sent her home. Two days later, when her temperature failed to drop, she went to a different hospital, where a second doctor took an X-ray of Miss Tsui's lungs and gave her some antibiotics. However, he told her that she had the common flu and nothing more. She then stayed home and did not meet anyone, not even the clients; all the same, a few days later she called her Singapore office to say she was returning home as she was not feeling well.

Her flight arrived at Changi Airport's terminal 1 at 5:38 a.m. The airport was beginning to implement a series of screening procedures advised by the WHO, but despite the new heightened state of alertness, the sick woman passed through unchallenged. She was met by her mother, who took her by taxi to Singapore General Hospital's Accident & Emergency Department. From there she was sent by ambulance to Tan Tock Seng Hospital—and diagnosed as having SARS.

* * *

By now it was clear that Tsui Mei-ling, now seriously ill at Tan Tock Seng Hospital, was more than just the fourth person to bring the SARS virus into Singapore.

Hitherto, all of Singapore's SARS patients could be traced to the first three women who brought the coronavirus home after visiting Hong Kong, and authorities were hoping that they had effectively thrown a quarantine cordon around them and everyone who had been in contact with them. Tsui provided a new "index case," and sparked a new round of tracking everyone who came into contact with her while she was infectious because they might be at risk too.

The nine-member flight and cabin crew of China Southern Airlines Wednesday flight CZ 355 were quarantined, and health authorities were trying to trace all passengers as well as anyone who went near Miss Tsui that morning. So far, only 13 of the 49 passengers had been contacted, but a particular problem was the lowest-profile person in the chain: the taxi driver who had driven Tsui and her mother to the hospital.

Nobody could rule out the possibility that she could have contaminated the taxi with the virus, which at the time was thought to be able to survive outside the body for about three hours. Three hours is a long time for a taxi in a major city. The cab was starting to look like a moving Petri dish. Taxi companies were alerted to this fact on late Friday morning and at once began calling up their drivers and broadcasting messages on the taxis' satellite-based terminals for the driver to come forward, but to no avail. The authorities were unable to identify him, even though there was closed-circuit television footage of the taxi queue at the time when the two women may have boarded the cab, as the recording was too blurred. In addition, the company's satellite-tracking system did not record fares its cabs picked up. It would take about a month to trace the cabby from the meter records of its 11,000 taxis.

At the airport, meanwhile, screening was still extremely patchy. Reporters from the *Straits Times* found that passengers checking in at Singapore Airlines (SIA) and Qantas counters were greeted with placards displaying health questions, while some travelers boarding United Airlines and Cathay Pacific flights said they were asked if they had flu symptoms. Several airlines, such as SIA and Cathay Pacific, also said they were keeping close tabs on passengers from check-in to their destinations.

SIA cabin crew had been told to ask sick passengers to put on face masks, and to offer masks to those sitting near them. Also, a meal tray used by a sick passenger would be sealed in a plastic bag, and one of the toilets on the plane would be kept locked, to be used only by the sick person. Crew serving sick passengers would be expected to wear face masks and surgical gloves; a maximum of two crew members, instead of the usual four, would serve such passengers.

But counter staff at one Asian carrier said they had not received any directives. Staff at another airline said it would be too much work to question every passenger. Other counter staff were worried. They said they had wanted to wear masks, but were told to remove them because they looked "unprofessional," and might intimidate passengers.

The airport wasn't the only point of entry to cause headaches for the Health Ministry. Singapore is connected to mainland Malaysia by a causeway, across which 50,000 people a day commuted. Like the border between Guangzhou and Hong Kong, it was another of the vital, umbilical connections that would be highlighted by SARS.

On March 28, it was announced that a Malaysian student nurse working at Singapore's Tan Tock Seng Hospital had developed SARS symptoms. The causeway clearly posed an entirely new set of screening problems. A medical team was deployed to be on 24-hour standby at the Sultanah Aminah Hospital on the Malaysian side of the causeway should any SARS suspects be detected. Immigration and Customs personnel at the checkpoint were told to be on the lookout for travelers showing any signs of the disease, and if so, to alert the medical team immediately.

All the same, over the next few weeks there were signs of a certain tension between the two states: Singapore was the international gateway at which SARS was imported from East Asia, and every so often news reports carried an underlying sense that Malays were starting to see their neighbors in a less open and friendly light.

At the beginning of April, the Malaysian Government advised the 50,000 Malaysians who commuted daily to work across the causeway to go on leave to avoid being infected. Malaya also began talking an increasingly tough line about Malays who persisted in visiting SARS-infected areas such as eastern China and Hong Kong. If they contracted SARS in those areas, a minister said, they might not be allowed back into Malaysia.

* * *

Another level at which quarantine was introduced—an especially important and problematic level—was within the Singapore healthcare system, and more specifically within the hospital system. The most significant step was the designation of one hospital—Tan Tock Seng—as the SARS treatment and isolation center. All but one wing of the sprawling hospital complex was closed, the patients transferred to hospitals elsewhere in the republic. All Tan Tock Seng staff were equipped with masks, gowns, and gloves. An air-conditioned tent was erected at the car park in front of the emergency room, where patients suspected of being infected with the disease were screened.

Help poured in from other public hospitals. KK Women's and Children's Hospital set up a children's ward at Tan Tock Seng when the first pediatric patients were identified. It sent four doctors and 18 nurses to staff it, and put another team of 11 nurses and six doctors on standby. It also sent child-sized ventilator masks and other equipment, even balloons and crayons.

With so many falling sick, the hospital ran out of isolation rooms. Fourteen rooms in an empty ward on level 13 were hastily converted. The air conditioning in the rooms was switched off and strong ventilation fans fitted to the windows, so the cool air from the corridors would be sucked into the rooms and vented outside. The ministry ordered 100,000 disposable plastic gowns and 130,000 masks. The hospital ordered more than 200,000 gloves, with other public hospitals sending supplies over until the orders arrived.

Staff were told to wear white T-shirts and baggy blue trousers instead of uniforms, for comfort and protection, and before leaving at the end of their shift, to shower and change into their own clothes, leaving the T-shirts and trousers to be laundered. Nobody was to care for a SARS patients without gown, mask, and gloves, and the gowns and gloves were to be disposed of before the staff member left the patient's room. The hospital bought several dozen germ warfare masks for use in high-risk procedures such as intubations. Despite these precautions, SARS spread. More than 100 staff also had their leave canceled, as more Tan Tock Seng staff fell ill. By mid-March, 37 staff had been diagnosed and another 10 admitted just in case.

It didn't take long for the public to know that medical personnel were at high risk for contracting SARS. Even before the schools were closed, principals asked several Tan Tock Seng staff to keep their children at home. One hospital worker said he was shunned by his relatives when he went to an uncle's funeral. Nurses in uniform riding the train found people shrinking away from them, and in one case a nurse who was seven months pregnant was asked to use the stairs rather than an elevator to get up to her seventh-floor apartment because she worked with SARS. This in itself was a kind of vigilante quarantine: isolation by association.

* * *

By Sunday, March 30, the Health Ministry had tracked down 30 of the 49 passengers who were with Miss Tsui on board the China Southern airlines flight from Beijing, but there was still no sign of the cab driver who had driven her and her mother from the airport to Singapore General Hospital. The 30 were found because they had given addresses in Singapore, and were ordered to stay home under quarantine law. The others had vanished, living testimony to the difficulty of tracking potential infectors, and the porousness of international borders.

Asked why it had taken so long to trace everyone connected with Miss Tsui, the National Environment Agency's head of quarantine and epidemiology, Dr. Goh Kee Tai, said they had difficulty even finding out from the sick woman and her mother what her flight number was.

As for the cab driver, the consensus theory was that the man wouldn't identify himself because he would be quarantined and lose 10 days' income. All three taxi companies—Comfort, CityCab and Tibs—said that said they would help the man financially if he was one of their employees. But the situation raised broader questions for the cabbies. What if the stigma, or the disease itself, infected all taxi drivers, and people shunned taxi rides in future? The anxiety went the other way as well: taxi drivers were becoming increasingly aware of the infection risks they faced. Many started to avoid taking passengers to Tan Tock Seng Hospital and its vicinity. Others began airing their cars after every trip, while a handful prepared masks which they might use if ferrying a sick passenger.

The close confines of a taxi, the contact with international travelers going to and from the airport, the randomness and under-the-radar profile all made that cab seem like a small bioweapon by itself.

* * *

The world of sports, a perfect setting to transmit disease, was also affected. The Hong Kong Rugby Sevens, going on the same time, turned out to be a strange event. The players performed in front of huge crowds of up to 30,000, but the events were overshadowed by SARS. "The headline in the paper," said Gary Tan, the men's team captain, "was 'Virus claims its 12th victim.' Next to it was a picture of Kenya beating Australia."

Off the field, the Singapore men's and women's teams were under strict rules. The 28 players and officials were confined to their hotel, training ground, and stadium. "There was minimal contact between teams," Tan said. "The Hong Kong captain had to call me in my room to ask whether we could swap jerseys. Even for the farewell dinner, it was dinner and then straight back to the hotel rooms. For our team, it was even stricter. We did not even step out onto the street."

When the two teams returned, 21 players and officials of the men's and women's teams were taken immediately to an undisclosed location for a week of quarantine, apparently at the request of their families. The remaining seven went home, where they were ordered to remain under house quarantine for a week.

The Hong Kong Sevens, though, didn't pass untainted. One of the Fiji players developed suspicious symptoms, and the next international rugby tournament, due to be held in Singapore a week later, was canceled. Sporting events in general were falling like bowling pins. The scheduled Commonwealth Bodybuilding Championships was postponed until July, after Malaysia and the Maldives pulled out. Silat, a martial art, was also affected: the national team was not sent to defend its title in Belgium because of the SARS scare.

"We heard that Belgium is very concerned about SARS, and might quarantine people who come from Singapore," the national coach, Sheikh Alauddin, said. "If that happens, we would have traveled for nothing."

* * *

A week after the quarantine orders were first handed out, 945 people were in home quarantine, including 38 entire families, 427 students, seven airport workers who had contact with Tsui Mei-ling, and 305 Motorola staff ordered to stay home after one of their colleagues went down with SARS.

The concept of isolating SARS patients within the hospitals, or sending them to a single containment and treatment site, turned out to be an oversimplification, as the virus began to spread around the hospitals, disguised under the symptoms of other illnesses.

Aliyah Mohammed (not her real name), 52, a mother of three and an employee of the Public Utilities Board, was warded in Tan Tock Seng Hospital on March 10 with bacterial pneumonia. She also had a long list of existing medical conditions—diabetes, hypertension, and other heart problems. She was admitted to a general ward, where she contracted the SARS virus from a nurse. Over the next few days she passed the virus on to a relative, three visitors, a fellow patient, and about 16 hospital staff. When she was later moved to the cardiac unit for her heart problems, she infected two physicians, one of them a cardiology trainee. The relative in turn infected her mother and four siblings. When Ms. Mohammed developed a fever, she was moved to the hospital's intensive care unit, where she lapsed into a coma and died after about five days. Several days later, Ong Hok Su, the 27-year-old doctor who had cared for her also died.

The Health Ministry had instructed all SARS victims to be cremated, but Muslims were an exception: Ms. Mohammed's body was buried, but sealed in two body bags to prevent the virus from escaping—her final form of quarantine.

* * *

A major labor issue arose from the very beginning of the outbreak: should quarantined workers be paid? The Ministry of Manpower, with input from the National Trades Union Congress, the Singapore Business Federation, and the Singapore National Employers Federation, drew up a set of guidelines for payroll managers, urging employers to accommodate people who chose to stay away from work on their own accord and parents who needed leave to tend to their children now that schools and child care centers had been shut.

On the other hand, the money had to come from somewhere, and the quarantine was now beginning to weigh on the calculations of local businesses. (Early in the Toronto outbreak a number of businesses refused to let workers go into quarantine because their absence would cost the owner money. Public health officials politely pointed out the relative cost of not sending the worker home and having an outbreak in the workplace, after which quarantine absence was granted a lot more readily.) The Ministry also asked employers to deduct quarantined workers' days of absence from their hospitalization leave entitlement, so that they could continue to be paid. If workers had used up this entitlement, it asked bosses to exercise "flexibility and compassion" in granting additional leave.

Bosses who sent workers home could let them clear their annual leave. Alternatively, they could work out an agreement with them. Either way, the bottom line was that these workers should continue getting at least half, if not their full, wages. Referring to the outbreak euphemistically as "a new experience," union chief Lim Boon Heng said: "We are learning of the ramifications day by day."

* * *

University students, who had initially been placed in an older-and-wiser category and excluded from the general quarantine imposed on institutions of education, were asked to disclose if they had traveled to countries affected by SARS. Being a mobile (and somewhat prone to feeling invulnerable) population, it was a matter of time before SARS crept into this group as well. Sure enough, despite the risk of SARS, some had been to China, Hong Kong, or Viet Nam. Of those who did so, the Singaporean students were sent into home quarantine, while foreign students were isolated in separate hostel rooms. They were all told to see the university doctors.

Later, university students returning from SARS-affected countries would be ordered to come back three weeks before the semester started in order to undergo quarantine.

* * *

The missing cabbie at last came forward—or rather, a cab driver came forward who remembered carrying a sick woman. It wasn't indisputably clear that this was, in fact, the right man, and the driver himself said he hoped he wasn't; but for his honesty he was given a quarantine order. Comfort, his company, said they would do their best to help: he wouldn't have to pay the rent of his vehicle during his quarantine and the company was willing to find ways to provide for any financial needs.

The taxi-driver scare revealed another crucial aspect of the quarantine: What to do about public transport, another perfect vector for a communicable disease? One tactic adopted by Singapore's Health Ministry was to try to reduce the need for actual or potential SARS victims to use buses and trains. They actually set aside a designated fleet of 32 ambulances for anyone who started displaying SARS symptoms while on quarantine at home, travelers from SARS areas who felt unwell, and those referred by general practitioners and dentists. People identified as SARS suspects during screening at Changi Airport and the cruise centre would also get an ambulance ride direct to Tan Tock Seng Hospital, the SARS center.

* * *

In both Defoe's Journal of the Plague Year and Albert Camus' La Peste (The Plague) the daily numbers count takes on an almost ritual identity, the figures themselves becoming the subject of intense scrutiny, interpretation, and prognostication. Singapore was no different. Newspapers began running daily totals, for example:

> Total infected 78
> In stable condition in hospital 49
> Seriously ill, in intensive care 11
> Discharged 16
> Dead 2

At the beginning of April 2003, Singapore suffered its fifth SARS death, and the total number with the disease surpassed 100—but there were only 32 still in hospital, the lowest in two weeks. The Health Minister remained cautious, saying the fight was not yet over and, with 13 people seriously ill, there could be more deaths. By April 5, the number of people still under home quarantine orders was 196, also apparently falling, but within days it was up to 260, and a single act of quarantine a few days later shot the total over 2,000. Numbers meant something, no doubt, but when all was said and done, the only important number to watch for was zero.

* * *

One aspect of Singapore's quarantine that raised eyebrows in the West was the fact that the promised "SARS task force," which would both enforce the quarantine and sustain the needs of those quarantined, consisted in part of a private police force. Cisco, Singapore's largest private security company, was brought in on April 10 after several people breached their quarantine orders. The work load immediately multiplied.

"We were told to expect 70 to 80 orders each day," Alvin Seng, its deputy director of protection and enforcement services, told the *Straits Times*. "Then. . . for our first assignment, we received 235 orders. We were shocked." By May 10, Cisco employees had issued 6,000 home quarantine orders, and fitted electronic bracelets on nine quarantine breakers. They had also installed video cameras in the homes of violators, who were instructed to appear before the cameras at specific times during the day.

In addition to the enforcement work, Cisco staff made visits with nurses to explain the order and the backup help available, phoned quarantinees between three and five times a day, and were often involved in making home deliveries of supplies.

Apart from "a handful" of people who slammed their doors when the Cisco officers turned up, many Singaporeans were remarkably cordial and hospitable when the security forces arrived. "Two to three out of every 10 offered me a drink," reported Sergeant Lim, "which I declined because I was in uniform."

Clearly, using private security officers to sustain quarantine creates a very different civic impact than using public health workers, yet even here the issues are not as clear as they might seem. Singapore is one of the wealthier places on the globe. It's not clear whether the city of Toronto could have afforded to hire a private security force to sustain its quarantine even if it had wanted to. By drafting in public health workers, the city was perhaps adopting the only affordable course of action—though that in turn meant that public health services in every walk of life and every area of the city suffered.

* * *

The assumption that Singapore's hospitals had worked out effective containment procedures was rudely shattered when it was discovered in early April that 20 nurses and a doctor from Singapore General Hospital were suffering from fevers and had to be classified as SARS suspects.

Another round of tracking and quarantine had to begin at once. Doctors suspected a patient who had had gastrointestinal bleeding, a kidney abscess, and a fever from a bacterial infection, not the expected symptoms of SARS—another instance of symptom camouflage.

About 70 patients in two wards were denied visitors, as health authorities attempted to reach around 500 people who had had contact with the sick doctors and nurses.

An especially frightening leak was feared when a nurse from the KK Women's and Children's Hospital was classified as a probable SARS case, because at the time some 500 pregnant women were in the hospital. More than 430 of the women were hastily contacted and checked, and luckily all seemed to be fine.

* * *

Health care settings produced two of the most intractable quarantine problems. One was that the virus was striking most effectively and widely within hospitals, which meant that the people most likely to be quarantined were those most vital in the fight against the virus. It seemed quite possible that within a couple of weeks, if quarantine were to be enforced among medical staff, there would be nobody left to care for the sick.

Toronto tried to deal with this issue by inventing "work quarantine."

"We invented—I think we invented—the concept of work quarantine," Bonnie Henry said wryly, "because we recognized [that even with so many health care workers sick] we still had to take care of patients. We had health care workers who were in quarantine at home, and they were allowed only to come to work. So they got the worst of both worlds. The hospital was a live environment. Every encounter at all times required the use of an N-95 mask, gloves, handwashing, et cetera. It was not a very pleasant experience for them."

The other problem was perhaps more surprising: doctors and nurses, it turned out, made up a high percentage of quarantine-breakers. One of the most egregious examples was a physician who broke quarantine to play tennis—with a reporter from one of the major local newspapers! The reporter, who must have wrestled with a tough ethical quandary, turned his tennis partner in, and the physician was one of the few who were issued a follow-up compulsory quarantine order in Toronto.

This disobedience by medical workers was a curious phenomenon, and one that, as far as we are aware, has not been studied. It seems possible that health care staff believe that they are best able to monitor their own symptoms and be the best judges of their own health—certainly, the old saying of doctors making the worst patients seems to apply here. Unfortunately, the SARS outbreak proved time and again that this was quite true: many doctors badly— even fatally— misjudged how sick they really were.

* * *

What about Singapore's foreign workers? Business travelers and tourists may be the most visible international movement, but as many as 1,200 workers from SARS-affected countries worked in Singapore every month, mainly in the manufacturing, services, and construction industries.

Again, Singapore decided to be both firm and consistent: from April 11, foreigners from SARS-affected countries—China, Hong Kong, Taiwan, Viet Nam, and Canada were specified—who came to work in Singapore were ordered to undergo 10 days' quarantine before they could start on their jobs.

Clearly, this also required a certain amount of flow control, as the amount of available quarantine space was limited; there was also the question of the cost to the employer. Singapore's government decided that batches of between 100 and 200 new work-permit holders would be allowed in at a time, and each would be put in dormitories at their employers' expense. The dormitories to house incoming work-permit holders had rooms about the size of a three-room Housing Board flat, and each room could house up to 10 people. Food was delivered to prevent them from mingling in the canteen with the existing 2,000 or so foreign workers there. They also got periodic medical checks. Employers had to pay about $350 for each worker's 10-day dormitory stay as well as medical expenses, which could amount to $80 per worker. Professionals and executives underwent home quarantine.

Once a guest worker returned to his or her home country, the quarantine would have to be repeated. A spokesman at Hua Kok International, a construction firm that hired about 130 workers from China, said: "If workers want to go home, we can't stop them. If they insist, we may consider asking them to pay the quarantine fee."

Singapore chose not to completely bar workers coming from these places because companies might require their expertise, said Manpower Minister Lee Boon Yang. "If you take the approach of building a wall around Singapore," Dr. Lee said, "at the end of the day, you might find that everything comes to a standstill."

* * *

It was only a matter of time before someone flagrantly and repeatedly ignored the quarantine, which until the second week of April had been essentially voluntary, despite the video cameras and the threat of fines. Would the government enforce the fines? And if the threat wasn't working, how would the quarantine be enforced?

On April 10, Health Minister Lim Hng Kiang told a press conference that 12 people had flouted their quarantine orders—five secondary and kindergarten students, one polytechnic student, and six immediate family members of SARS patients. They had been found out because they did not answer calls from the health officials checking on them, or were not at home when spot checks were carried out.

In one case, a woman under stay-home orders came down with a fever and went to see her doctor without revealing she was under quarantine. Two days later, when her fever had not gone down, her relatives broke their quarantine and ferried her in a car to the National University Hospital, instead of using the ambulance service to Tan Tock Seng. She became too ill to be transferred, and was moved to the intensive care unit. Her husband, too, developed SARS, though nobody else who came into contact with the family seemed affected.

Minister Lim, visibly upset, commented, "This irresponsible behavior presents not just a risk to the public but can also cause other hospitals to become contaminated with SARS." From now on, he said, a new system of surveillance would be put in place, not just for the scofflaws but for all 490 people currently under quarantine: officers at once began installing cameras in the quarantine homes, and when health care workers called, a quarantined person must switch on the camera and stand in front of it. If he or she was not at home when the health care worker called to check, the result would be a written warning, and the offender would have to wear an electronic surveillance bracelet like those used by prisoners on furlough.

Three repeat offenders would actually find themselves forced to wear these bracelets before April was out.

* * *

The fear of SARS had a silver lining for the Pizza Hut and Kentucky Fried Chicken chains: with people staying at home more often, the food-delivery business saw a double-digit percentage growth in the first month of the quarantine. But here, too, was another possible disease vector: the pizza delivery boy as superinfector. Interestingly, the need for home-delivered food seems to have been more potent than the fear of the delivery boy on one's doormat—though in some cases, at least, the delivery companies made their employees wear masks as well.

* * *

A week after SARS was first discovered at Singapore General, the disease had broken out of the two wards into which it was thought confined.

Two people, a patient and a visitor, died. The Urology Outpatient Centre, the diagnostic radiology area, and the radiology archives were closed. The hospital quarantined 120 staff working at the urology and radiology departments, as well as 279 patients.

After the first group of patients and staff were moved out, Singapore General said the workload of 45 affected general surgeons would be done by its urologists and colorectal surgeons. With Urology closed, the 10 colorectal surgeons had to bear the full load—but that was less of a burden than it might appear, as the hospital had stopped all nonemergency operations.

Two days later, the National Cancer Centre shut down its radiology department when a radiographer and a porter were diagnosed with SARS. About 200 patients had to be traced and 47 people placed on home quarantine. The importance of both the tracking and quarantine aspects of the crisis was underscored when another SARS patient died—a woman in her forties who violated her home quarantine twice, once to see her family doctor, instead of going to Tan Tock Seng Hospital as required by the order, and again to get a relative, also under home quarantine, to drive her to National University Hospital for treatment.

The public's sympathy with the quarantine measures was by no means uniform. Visitors to hospitals were distressed, distraught, or outraged that they weren't allowed to see their loved ones, and didn't always recognize that the restrictions were for their own good. Health care workers at several hospitals reported that they had been cursed at and nearly beaten up for turning visitors away if they looked feverish, tried to sneak in back doors, or attempted to intimidate the staff.

* * *

As time passed, it began to seem as if the quarantine was no single entity, but a series of individual cases cropping up all over the city like the virus itself. Rule by fiat began to seem not so much a violation of civil liberties as an oversimplification: whatever the general public health principles, it was far easier to make a decree than to work out how to apply it in every possible case.

Saudi Arabia banned visitors from Singapore, preventing at least 45 Singaporean Muslims from going on pilgrimage to Mecca. When an employee of the Pasir Panjang vegetable market fell sick, police vans and cars blocked the entrance, closing down the 1,000 stalls. More than 2,000 of the sick man,s co-workers were quarantined, and officials at the border turned back five trucks of produce from Malaysia because the drivers had recently made deliveries to the Singapore market.

In the aftermath of the outbreak—and in a grim foreshadowing of the slaughter of civets in China nearly a year later—the Agri-Food and Veterinary Authority (AVA) began a program to sterilize and cull (that is, catch and kill) stray cats, especially those found around markets. At one point the cull was taking in 45 cats a day. The AVA denied this had anything to do with SARS, but animal lovers were skeptical, and some began rounding up strays and sending them to an animal shelter. Tests of blood and stool samples of the cats for the SARS virus were inconclusive. Screening at Changi Airport became steadily more rigorous—so much so that the Taiwanese rock band Mayday, in Singapore to play a benefit concert, decided to abandon the face masks they had brought along. The surveillance process was ratcheted up a degree a week later when the airport installed thermal scanners—modified military equipment designed to identify heat sources at night—intended to pick up heat traces from anyone running a fever. All the same, airport traffic was reported to have fallen more than 10 percent, with more attrition expected.

A Comfort Cab driver, ferrying passengers to the hospital, did indeed contract SARS, and again the tracking process went into high gear. The three taxicab companies decided to set up 12 stations around Singapore where drivers could stop by to have their temperature checked. Drivers began driving with their windows down and the air conditioning off to help keep the air in the cab fresh—albeit warm.

On April 26, the government and opposition MPs closed ranks to pass still more stringent quarantine laws, effective immediately; laws that in retrospect expressed frustration as much as legislative planning. Quarantine breakers could be jailed for six months and fined $10,000 even for a first offense. Property could be isolated and even demolished to prevent the spread of infection, a likely response to the Amoy Gardens situation. Anyone who even suspected he or she was infectious and left home nevertheless could be punished, as could anyone who gave false information or refused to cooperate.

To the world at large, these seemed like extreme measures. The *Toronto Star* described quarantined Singaporeans as "under virtual house arrest" and the wrist tags as "even more intrusive surveillance." A columnist in the *Straits Times* responded, "[I]f this government chooses to be 'draconian' in this instance, so be it. Because all it takes is one person or just a handful to be blissfully ignorant or deliberately defiant, and we're down the slippery slope."

It's also important to note that these were only the most aggressive and globally publicized means of prevention. SARS information and prevention advice in Singapore increased rapidly, using various types of media. These, including the disease's very own outlet, the "SARS Channel," were established to give current and comprehensive information on world infection trends and Singapore's situation. The Ministry of Health provided SARS information on its website, taking advantage of the fact that Singapore is a remarkably wired community: roughly two-thirds of its population was on the Internet.

* * *

While these new measures were being passed, in many respects the initial anxiety and upheaval was beginning to calm down, and by mid-April at least some aspects of Singapore life were returning to normal. SARS might not be suppressed, but people had learned to adapt and live with it, or at least with the fear of it. A 34-year-old pilot with Transmile Air Cargo was hospitalized with SARS in Malaysia, having picked up the virus at the airport hotel in Hong Kong. Two months previously, this would have been the world's nightmare—a pilot carrying the pandemic from country to country. Now it meant running through an established routine, with contacts to be tracked down and quarantined. On a more mundane level, children were going back to school and to neighborhood playgrounds, the downtown stores and shopping malls were no longer deserted. And perhaps the surest sign of recovery, commercial validation of the situation: a fitness company was offering a SARS deal, to buy a stationary bicycle or treadmill and get a thermometer and one month's supply of masks free.

* * *

In the end, only one person was charged and convicted of breach of quarantine. Chua Hock Seng, quarantined on April 29, was twice found to be not at home when Cisco officers called, and later went out drinking and made the strategic error of showing off his quarantine order. The other patrons around him, alarmed, called for an ambulance that took him to Ten Tock Seng Hospital—but two days later he did the same thing again. He was arrested, and in a very public show of resolve, the Prime Minister called his behavior "madness," the Home Affairs Minister announced that Chua would be "dealt with," and the Minister of State called the behavior "totally unacceptable." He was given the maximum penalty of six months in jail. The judge told him, "Your conduct. . . is irresponsible and incorrigible. In fact, given the current situation, it is reckless conduct because it puts the unsuspecting public and public health at risk." Four months in jail would be the starting point for most first offenders, but Chua received the maximum jail term because he had a long list of previous convictions for disorderly behavior and injuring others with weapons.

* * *

Just as the outbreak in Singapore was winding down, events in Taiwan threw the entire question of quarantine into a new light. On April 22, 2003, Taiwan had 29 probable cases, no deaths and a slow growth rate—typical of a minor outbreak. However, a new cluster of seven infections in Hoping Hospital in Taipei was reported on that day. This started a chain of transmission that led to 116 probable cases and 10 deaths in two weeks. In the days that followed, the numbers grew to 264 cases and 34 deaths by mid-May, and 680 cases and 81 deaths by June 1—more than a sixfold increase in less than a month. As the tension rose to near panic levels in Taiwan, the health authorities tried to enforce house quarantine of tens of thousands of persons, mainly those with contacts to the suspected case-patients and to arrivals from affected areas abroad, but the quarantine was broken repeatedly. Interestingly, though, SARS spread not so much from breach of quarantine but in the hospitals—even at this late stage in the epidemic, when hospital precautions had already become fairly well developed. This observation bears repeating: SARS was more likely to spread in a hospital than because of quarantine breakers.

One study subsequently suggested that the key factor in the spread was triage—in other words, how accurately and rapidly patients went from the possible SARS category to the probable. Someone at home with early-stage SARS turns out to be very unlikely to infect even close family members and friends; someone in hospital with more advanced SARS, especially if the disease is undiagnosed and the isolation is lax, is potentially the most dangerous player in a SARS outbreak. Quarantine, the Taiwan experience suggested, was an important but secondary means of preventing a SARS epidemic.

Other studies were also emerging by now. One found that more than 80 percent of the public thought official information was accurate, clear, sufficient, timely, and trustworthy, and 72 percent were prepared to accept a 10-day quarantine, even in the absence of SARS symptoms or close contact with a SARS patient. Other studies in Hong Kong and Toronto, on the other hand, found a high incidence of post-traumatic stress disorder symptoms and depression among quarantinees, and some variable rates of compliance: 86 percent of quarantined persons wore a mask in the presence of household members; but only 58 percent remained inside their residence for the duration of their quarantine. Thirty-three percent of those quarantined did not monitor their temperatures as recommended: 26 percent self-monitored their temperatures less frequently than recommended, and 7 percent did not measure their temperatures at all. Quarantine was, and probably always will be, a fallible tool.

Whereas SARS badly shook the public's faith in government in China and Hong Kong, the reverse was true in Singapore, the study suggested: "it corroborated the usefulness of public health and environmental regulations" and conversely demonstrated "a relatively high level of social discipline in the population."

Yet the issue of public obedience was clearly not so simple. Another study found that 60 percent of Singaporeans wanted to be told if one of their neighbors had been served with a home quarantine order, yet only one in three said they would tell their neighbors if they themselves were quarantined. Anxiety and stigma were clearly major issues that were never fully resolved.

* * *

As May progressed, with no new cases reported one day, then the next, the quarantine seemed to be holding. If there were no new cases for 20 days, the WHO had said, it would remove a country from its list of those affected by SARS. Viet Nam was already off the list. Could Singapore be next? Just hours ahead of the deadline, a 30-year-old surveyor, having his temperature taken during the morning screening at his construction site office, was found to be running a fever and hospitalized. Several colleagues were quarantined, and the office disinfected.

Yet that was the virus's last card. On May 31, a day ahead of the required 20-day period, WHO announced that Singapore was being taken off its list of SARS-affected countries. David Heymann thanked the people of Singapore "for your excellent collaboration these past months."

Since arriving in March, SARS had infected 206 people, of whom 31 had died. Nine people were still in the hospital, four of them critically ill.

A spokesman for the Ministry of Health reminded Singaporeans to "continue to maintain the highest level of vigilance. The possibility of a future imported case sparking off clusters of SARS cases in Singapore cannot be discounted," he said, making a veiled reference to Toronto, which was removed from the WHO list but then returned to it 12 days later. "So long as there are SARS-affected areas in the region and the world, we cannot afford to let our guard down."

* * *

After the outbreak was over, it was a common observation that perhaps more people had been quarantined than necessary.

A couple of conclusions seem worth making. First, at the beginning of the outbreak, and especially when the Amoy Gardens outbreak occurred, it was very hard to say with confidence how far SARS would spread, and how fast. Erring on the safe side may have caused more social disruption than necessary, and certainly more social disruption than could have been foreseen, but it was probably widespread.

Second, quarantine turned out to be the flip side of contact tracing, which in turn was intimately connected with the degree of transparency among public health officials. In places where the outbreak was acknowledged and taken seriously at once, contact tracing could begin straight away and the result could be a selective and targeted quarantine. The later the contact tracing began, the less precise it could be, and the wider the quarantine net had to be thrown. China was forced, in effect, to quarantine whole cities, and to threaten the sternest penalties for violation. SARS showed that some degree of quarantine is probably always necessary, but mass quarantine is a weapon of last resort.

Chapter 16.

People Would Move Away: SARS and Stigma

One of the less attractive features of human nature is that when we are afraid we look for someone to blame for our fear.

In an outbreak of infectious disease this leads to the pathogen being personified and demonized ("killer bug"), but a nonsentient, all-but-invisible entity makes a poor culprit. The best candidates for blame are humans who in some respect seem to have brought the killer bug closer to ourselves or to those we care about. In an epidemic of infectious disease, the best way to spread the pathogen is to be infected oneself; as such, SARS offered constant and worldwide opportunities for blaming the victim.

Governments led a generalized stigma by rushing out legislation denying visas, jobs, or even entry to anyone from SARS-affected countries. This, as pointed out previously, went far beyond the WHO's recommendation, which was to screen travelers and identify those who were actually (or possibly) sick. The entry bans based on nationality or origin were the equivalent of the slaughter of every chicken in Hong Kong.

This reflexive counterattack in turn led to a general West-versus-East prejudice familiar in flu season, where East Asia is conversationally blamed for being the birthplace of wave upon wave of influenza viruses. In the early days of the outbreak, a number of newspapers quoted medical pundits who explicitly blamed the atypical pneumonia cases on the primitive standards of living in South China, where people were supposed to be living cheek-by-jowl with pigs and chickens, and also by implication on the poor standard of East Asian health care. One of the unfortunate effects of China's early refusal to communicate openly about the outbreak (which gave Western editorialists the opportunity for some spectacularly unfettered China-bashing) was that nobody in the

West knew how well Chinese physicians had already characterized the disease and recommended suitable treatment.

Garry Smyth, traveling from Switzerland to East Asia during the epidemic, discovered these attitudes at first hand. Not only was the situation less frightening than he'd been led to believe, but the quality of healthcare was superb. "These are very up-to-date, well-run, modern hospitals. Yet the word on the street in Europe or North America was, 'Man, why are you doing that? You're going to your death.'"

In this climate of distrust and prejudice, anyone from Hong Kong was likely to be shunned, even by intelligent people, even by health professionals. Professor Mary Waye of the Chinese University of Hong Kong had been invited to deliver a paper in Germany and then go on to a symposium at Cambridge University to mark the 50th anniversary of the discovery of DNA. She was suddenly very aware of coming from Hong Kong. In her hotel in Germany, she noticed that nobody else seemed to have been assigned a room near hers. In England, she had been invited to a party, but at the last moment got a phone call to disinvite her. It took conscious acts of social initiative to begin to dispel the stigma. When someone uneasily asked Richard Henderson, her host in Cambridge, whether it was true that someone from Hong Kong was coming to the symposium, he answered, "Yes, and she's staying at my house."

* * *

Once the word got out that the infection was spreading mostly in hospitals all over the world, health care workers were treated not as heroes but as carriers.

"The initial stages were painful for our staff," said Dr Brenda Ang of Tan Tock Seng Hospital, echoing stories that were also commonplace in Hong Kong, Toronto, and elsewhere, "because they faced a lot of fear and discrimination from the public. We had many, many cases of our nurses who if they were to leave in their uniforms would not be able to get a cab. Buses would not stop for them, and if they were on the subway, trying to get a seat, the rest of the people would move away. We had reports of schools or educational centers... stopping children from our staff from going to school."

"But I think the general feeling has turned around quite dramatically. The public and the rest of Singapore moved away from the fear and discrimination to one of, at first, sympathy and then outright support. Of course, that was helped tremendously by [the fact that] the full Ministry, Cabinet, and the whole country basically turned around. That is why you see all these cards and measures of support, so much so that every day we have free cakes at lunch plus free flowers. That has helped tremendously."

We don't know of any systematic study that has explained why this turnaround took place, but it seems to have been helped by two elements: the public's confidence in their government, and the role of the media in helping to support a tone of support. Media studies of the SARS outbreak are in their infancy, but it's clear that an alarmist media is likely to be divisive. In Singapore in particular, the *Straits Times* was notable for its willingness to get in among patients, public health workers, hospital staff, and members of the public and depict the ongoing events as a human story, rather than a political football or a series of horrifying crises.

SARS contacts in quarantine were avoided to a degree that often crossed over from caution into absurdity and paranoia. Individuals and groups in schools, apartment buildings, or in hostels (where it became known that people had been put into quarantine) were systematically shunned. In Toronto, there were reports of apartment block and condominium residents demanding that new parking arrangements be made so they didn't have to park their cars next to the cars of people in quarantine.

While some prejudicial views were the result of straightforward anxiety—people's reluctance to eat in Chinese restaurants during the outbreak, for example—others were more complicated. In Toronto, one neighborhood of Russians felt stigmatized by location and history. An apartment block with two cases of SARS happened to be home to a large number of Russian families, who discovered that pizza shops wouldn't deliver and the phone company wouldn't do repairs. They began to think they were being discriminated against not just because of their location, but because of their ethnic identity. Many of the Russian-Canadians were also a little hostile to TPH: having suffered through years of being lied to by the government in their native land, they were inclined to be suspicious of TPH in an example of what might be called reverse stigmatization.

Perhaps the saddest and most brutal acts of prejudice concerned the Bukas-Loob Sa Diyos Filipino catholic community in Toronto.

As soon as it became clear that multiple infections had taken place among them, the press took to referring to them as a "sect" or even a "cult," inspiring suspicion rather than sympathy, and the group quarantine had the effect of creating a collective stigma. In point of fact, the quarantine was exceptionally hard on the members of the Bukas-Loob Sa Diyos, to whom community had an especially important meaning; they were more like an extended family than a congregation, and to be separated from each other caused great distress. In addition, many of them were self-employed, so the quarantine caused financial hardship. Some who worked as nannies suffered a particularly cruel fate: not only were they forced to lose work, but in some instances their family employers didn't want them to come back.

The blame-the-victim spirit was also alive and well in Hong Kong. One recovered SARS patient told the Health Department's fact-finding committee: "I am no longer working. I have left my company because my company regarded SARS patients unfavorably. . . . I live in a very small neighborhood; my wife was a saleslady there. Everybody in the neighborhood knew about my contracting the illness, and she was also discriminated against, and we had a hard time."

Another recovered SARS patient added: "A lot of people in the community had fear about contracting the virus because of inadequate knowledge about the disease. My wife was given a warning letter from her company because she had to take care of me, and her salary also got cut because of that."

Residents of Amoy Gardens were, bluntly put, treated like lepers of old. Some of their employers forbade them to come to work even though they were not infected, and the phrase "from Amoy Gardens" became shorthand for "infected with the SARS virus." This was true even among health care workers in SARS wards who themselves were feeling discriminated against: "It seemed that all our colleagues in the ward were regarded as infectious patients. Even when we took the lift or went to the canteen, despite the fact that we had washed our hands and taken the precautions, others treated us like the residents of Amoy Gardens. Our colleagues turned away from us and we felt very lonely. . . . "

These anxieties were repeated all over the world, even where there was no outbreak to speak of. In the United States, the situation was especially delicate on the West Coast, with its sizeable Asian population.

When Annie Yang, an 18-year-old from California, went to the airport to meet her mother, returning from a trip to China, she found herself covering her mouth with her hand. Her mother subsequently did, in fact, develop pneumonia, but not of the SARS variety; all the same, when she came home from the hospital Annie's friends were scared to visit. Her mother was taking an adult education class, and when fellow students heard that she had recently come home sick from China, they called the director of the classes to demand that she not be allowed to return to class until she brought proof that she had not been infected with SARS.

A 27-year-old engineer from San Jose came back from Hong Kong, Thailand, and Vietnam and decided to quarantine himself just in case, but people were not mollified.

``People are paranoid," he said. "My parents didn't want to see me for like a week."

Visits to Canada were also likely to create stigma and provoke anxiety. After an Ohio school band returned from Toronto, "five or six" worried parents called the school, and even though none of the children showed any sign of infection, and the CDC in Atlanta apparently recommended otherwise, the school was closed "as a precaution."

In England, anxiety about SARS led several private schools in Britain to bar students returning from spring break in Singapore, Hong Kong, and China's Guangdong province. Some children stayed in hotels with their parents, others were diverted to Ireland, Holland, and France, and 155 went to quarantine camps in Dorset and the Isle of Wight.

The headmaster of a boarding school in Blackpool, in northern England, arranged to rent one wing of a hotel in Blackpool for the children to remain in an unofficial quarantine for a week. They were to be supervised by a nurse, separated from the rest of the guests, and to receive their meals by room service. When word got out, other guests formed what the *Times* called "an abusive mob" and insisted the management throw the children out at once. For his pains, the unfortunate headmaster saw his face on the front page of a newspaper, captioned:

"THE MAN WHO BROUGHT SARS TO BLACKPOOL".

* * *

Dealing with stigmatization came disturbingly low on most nations' priorities, but some examples are worth looking at.

In theory, the hotlines run by most countries' public health systems and the follow-up calls made to people in quarantine were chances to offer support and encouragement. In Toronto, for example, a mental health nurse was always available on each floor of 277 Victoria, but the volume of calls made it hard to achieve much by phone.

Barbara Switzer in Toronto dealt with residents' fear of the Chinese community by holding an education-and-support meeting for residents of an apartment complex and then leading everyone across the road to have dinner at a Chinese restaurant. Likewise, on April 10, Prime Minister Jean Chrétien dined at a Chinese restaurant in Toronto in an effort to dispel fears about SARS.

On a larger scale, the entire city of Toronto tried to dispel fears about SARS by staging a six-hour downtown Concert For Toronto featuring an all-Canadian lineup, including Avril Lavigne, The Barenaked Ladies, Sarah McLachlan, The Tragically Hip, and Diana Krall.

In fact, anything that shows life going on as usual can be said to combat the effects of stigma, though any such activity can also potentially pose risks, both clinical and psychological. The Hong Kong Sevens rugby, for example, was a popular activity that showed how life in Hong Kong was still possible during the outbreak, and also kept the economy trickling through the province; yet the threat of infection meant that even the business-as-usual news coverage was saturated with news of precautions and the possibility of infection.

Perhaps the best illustration of the stigma of SARS is remarkable in its invisibility: room 911 at the Metropole Hotel no longer exists. Nowadays, guests step out of the elevator (the suspect elevator, the "vertical vector") on the ninth floor, past two framed Chinese prints, turn right and then pass room 913, then room 909. Room 911 is a victim of the virus, and the hotel as a whole has done its share of suffering. When the link between Professor Liu, Hong Kong, and the Metropole was discovered on March 19, 2003, panic set in among the guests, according to the South China Morning Post, "and an exodus from the 487-room hotel that left it deserted."

The stigma lingered even a year later. Several people who heard that I was staying at the Metropole (in 2004) told me I was braver than they would have been. However, two went on to add on reflection that now, after all that had happened, it's probably the cleanest and most hygienic hotel in Hong Kong. An article in the local paper on the anniversary of the virus reaching Hong Kong quoted the manager, indignantly upbeat, saying that the hotel was fully booked and unaffected by its history. This seemed a bit of a stretch: it didn't look fully booked to me, and I was able to extend my own booking for six days without the slightest problem.

* * *

In a sense, the issue of stigma is the flip side of the necessary acts of quarantine and isolation: any time someone was isolated, all the issues of blame, guilt, shame, anger, and resentment might arise. This was surely at its most agonizing for the dying and their families. A Canadian hospice worker told me how difficult it was during the SARS outbreak for both the dying and their relatives not to be able to see each other, let alone to hold a hand or stroke a forehead.

In June 2003, Elaine Lim, the woman who had been the index case for Singapore's outbreak, finally appeared in public on television. Both her parents and her pastor had caught SARS from her. Her father and the pastor later died, but she never saw them: she wasn't allowed out of isolation. Instead, she found herself being labeled a "super-infector," and blamed for the outbreak in Singapore.

She was finally allowed to return home in mid-April, according to Channel NewsAsia. "She now spends her time looking after her grandmother." To the world at large, these seemed like extreme measures. The *Toronto Star* described quarantined Singaporeans as "under virtual house arrest" and the wrist tags as "even more intrusive surveillance." A columnist in the *Straits Times* responded, "[I]f this government chooses to be 'draconian' in this instance, so be it. Because all it takes is one person or just a handful to be blissfully ignorant or deliberately defiant, and we're down the slippery slope."

It's also important to note that these were only the most aggressive and globally publicized means of prevention. SARS information and prevention advice in Singapore increased rapidly, using various types of media. These, including the disease's very own outlet, the "SARS Channel," were established to give current and comprehensive information on world infection trends and Singapore's situation. The Ministry of Health provided SARS information on its website, taking advantage of the fact that Singapore is a remarkably wired community: roughly two-thirds of its population was on the Internet.

* * *

While these new measures were being passed, in many respects the initial anxiety and upheaval was beginning to calm down, and by mid-April at least some aspects of Singapore life were returning to normal. SARS might not be suppressed, but people had learned to adapt and live with it, or at least with the fear of it. A 34-year-old pilot with Transmile Air Cargo was hospitalized with SARS in Malaysia, having picked up the virus at the airport hotel in Hong Kong. Two months previously, this would have been the world's nightmare—a pilot carrying the pandemic from country to country. Now it meant running through an established routine, with contacts to be tracked down and quarantined. On a more mundane level, children were going back to school and to neighborhood playgrounds, the downtown stores and shopping malls were no longer deserted. And perhaps the surest sign of recovery, commercial validation of the situation: a fitness company was offering a SARS deal, to buy a stationary bicycle or treadmill and get a thermometer and one month's supply of masks free.

* * *

Chapter 17.

Dire Straits: China and Taiwan

In the second half of March 2003, two forces were gathering strength in Beijing: an outbreak of SARS, largely unacknowledged, untraced, and uncontrolled, was spreading, and the World Health Organization was becoming more and more frustrated.

Because it is a United Nations' agency, and therefore only able to take part in investigations when invited by its host country, the WHO was in the difficult position of having a sizeable presence in Beijing that was involved in a number of public health campaigns and activities, but the SARS door was shut in its face. The early requests, in February and early March, for information and travel to Guangdong were stalled or turned down. As late as March 23, when a second special WHO team arrived in Beijing, the agency still didn't know whether, as it suspected, the reported atypical pneumonia in Guangdong had any connection to the disease now called SARS that was taking other countries, especially Hong Kong, by force. By the beginning of April, the team was in an impossible position: the WHO had just issued its first travel advisory for Guangdong, yet government officials were still telling the WHO team that the outbreak was under control.

Curiously, the problems in China were almost diametrically opposite to the way they were often depicted in the Western media, which saw a stubborn, old-fashioned communist central government refusing to admit the seriousness of the situation and to admit they could possibly have made mistakes.

In fact, the main difficulty, said Dr. Henk Bekedam, head of the WHO Beijing office, was how decentralized the country was. Governors of individual provinces had more authority in their own domains than the minister of health in Beijing—or, indeed, anyone in Beijing below the very highest levels of government.

Many of the issues that arose in China from trying to work across different areas of authority were actually similar to those found in Canada, he said, where "the sharing of information between the layers is not automatic."

"When China can use [authority at] the level of [Premier] Wen Jiabao," Bekedam said, "then China is again one China and they can do something very strongly. But from a governmental point of view it is rather decentralized... the government had to work very hard to convince the Guangdong authorities to accept us. That was a major breakthrough, to get to the province."

Arriving in Guangdong on April 3, the WHO team was impressed by the quality of the health care under tremendous pressure: during the second week of February, one hospital had 150 of its 400 beds devoted to SARS patients. Even so, surveillance and reporting were excellent, and the team was confident that any new cases would be detected and rapidly reported.

Elsewhere, though, there was cause for concern: Guangdong was the exception, rather than the rule, and most other provinces were poorer and less well equipped in every respect. Most disturbing of all, Beijing itself was vulnerable: "Only a minority of hospitals make daily reports of SARS cases," said the WHO report. "Contact tracing is another problem in Beijing and does not appear to be carried out systematically."

This in turn may have been news, strangely enough, to the Beijing government. Bekedam had the impression that information had crossed borders so slowly and awkwardly that at least some authorities in Beijing were so ill-informed that they genuinely thought that SARS was not much of a problem, and was in any case largely limited to Guangdong.

If that was the case, they were soon to hear otherwise.

By early April, the Chinese government was under increasing pressure from both within and without.

Jiang Yanyong, a senior surgeon at Beijing's Number 301 military hospital and a Communist Party member for 50 years, took the extraordinary step of publicly accusing Health Minister Zhang Wenkang of covering up the number of cases in Beijing. He said medical staff in Beijing's military hospitals were briefed about the dangers of SARS at the beginning of the National People's Congress in early March, but were told not to publicize what they'd learned lest it interfere with the annual meeting. Jiang said doctors at Beijing's No.

309 PLA Hospital told him they were treating 60 SARS patients and that seven patients had died of SARS.

Zhong Nanshan, director of the Respiratory Disease Research Institute in Guangzhou, said that the government's long-held view was neither objective nor based on medical analysis. "Looking at this from a medical point of view, this disease has not been effectively controlled at all, including in Hong Kong," he said at a briefing in Beijing. "The origin of this disease is still not clear, so how can you say it has been controlled?"

The WHO, meanwhile, was saying much the same to the Vice Premier, and other outside influences were making themselves felt. Emboldened and in some cases informed by whistleblowers like Dr. Jiang, Western newspapers ran almost daily exposés of attempts to falsify numbers or hide SARS patients. The *New York Times*, for example, published an account of the dire situation in Inner Mongolia:

"Meng Chunying says she felt the beginnings of a nasty head cold on March 18. But Ms. Meng, an Air China flight attendant who often flew the Hong Kong-Beijing route, said she never made the connection with an outbreak of atypical pneumonia that she thought was under control. A few days later, Ms. Meng, feeling listless and feverish, flew to Hohhot, the wind-swept capital of the Chinese region of Inner Mongolia, to see her family... she described the Hohhot Hospital as 'completely unprepared,' initially putting her into a room with patients who had different diseases. Mr. Li sat by her bedside day and night, never wearing a mask. They shared tea and steamed dumplings. Only in early April did doctors diagnose her SARS. When her husband, brother, and stepfather took ill, the hospital staff panicked and refused to treat them, Ms. Meng said. The hospital manager eventually relented and put them all in isolation in the burn ward. The disease had spread to health workers anyway. At the nearby Hohhot Chest Hospital, the main treatment center for lung diseases, SARS infected half a dozen medical workers. Frightened staff members refused to work, leaving the hospital critically short-handed. Huang Qi, the deputy general manager of the chest hospital, worked day and night in the SARS ward, even wheeling dead bodies to the 'peace room,' or morgue. Mr. Huang was later found to have SARS."

Another factor may have been that SARS began to penetrate even into the upper levels of the political and business hierarchy. Zhu

Hong, the deputy director of the department of trade and international affairs in the Commerce Ministry, took ill a few days after returning from a visit to Thailand, and Li Jikai, group executive director of the Chinese International Trust and Investment Corporation, or Citic, the leading state-owned industrial and financial conglomerate, also contracted SARS, according to the New York Times.

The *Times* added: "SARS even passed through the heavily guarded gates of Zhongnanhai, the exclusive leadership compound in the heart of the capital, infecting a maid who works for the widow of Chen Yun, family friends said. Mr. Chen, a veteran of the Long March who died in 1995, was long considered the only senior leader with influence to rival that of Deng Xiaoping, China's top leader from 1978 until his death in 1997." In a sign of the country's developing transparency, China's president Hu Jintao said on state television that he was "very worried" by SARS. The powerful Politburo Standing Committee held a special meeting on SARS, concluding with the statement, "There must be no delay and no deceit in reporting." Premier Wen Jiabao pledged China will "speak the truth" in disclosing facts and figures about SARS, and put the subject at the top of his cabinet's agenda twice in a week.

The WHO was also adding its weight, trying to impress on the government that releasing figures that lacked credibility was likely to damage not only China's standing internationally but might lead to domestic catastrophe. Based on the assessments made by the WHO team, Bekedam held a press conference to announce that, from the few hospitals the team had been allowed to inspect, he estimated that the number of deaths from SARS was "not thirty but at least two hundred."

The turning point came on April 20, 2003. The Health Minister, Zhang Wenkang, and the mayor of Beijing, Meng Xuenong (who had stated just days previously that Chinese health officials had "full control over atypical pneumonia"), were fired, followed shortly by several other senior officials including the Communist Party secretary, the director of the Center for Disease Control in Changsha, the capital of Hunan province, and three other officials in charge of disinfecting activities and running the city's SARS hotline. According to the Economist, Zhang Wenkang was the first minister since the Communists seized power in 1949 to be sacked mid-crisis on a policy matter.

This was the moment, Bekedam argued, when it finally became clear to everyone in China and all over the world that the central government was now fully engaged in the fight against SARS, and would override the provincial governments whenever necessary. The official number of SARS cases in the country was revised upward tenfold, to 339, and the government admitted that there might be hundreds more victims in hospitals or at home.

"We had hoped," Bekedam said, "that the initial increase of the cases was just because of the backlog"—in other words, these were people who had already been sick but had previously been uncounted. The city has over a hundred clinics, and the WHO team had only seen seven by this point, "but indeed it started massively spreading. I must stress, we had no idea where things were going. It was a time of great uncertainty."

Over the next few days Wen Jiabao announced the health system was so inadequate an epidemic could spread "before we know it" and "the consequences could be too dreadful to contemplate." The WHO warned that China might be facing a "very big outbreak" in the countryside, where resources were severely limited and where 70 percent of China's 1.3 billion people live. The government pledged more than $100 million for disease control in the poorest provinces. Wen called for an overhaul of the system for dealing with public medical emergencies and ordered a campaign to scrub down planes, trains, buses, taxis, and office blocks. All over the country, fever clinics were opened. One of the most massive and accelerated acts of public health in history was under way.

"Once they got on with the fight, I don't think there was any better country than China in dealing with it," Bekedam said. "One thing that China did, which would have been impossible in the United States or in my home country of the Netherlands, or in any Western country, was that in Beijing they told about 30 percent of the population to stand still and not move." Anyone who lived near a SARS case (this imprecision is a perfect illustration of what happens without accurate contact tracing) had to stay home for two to three weeks. "And they did it. And if you have an infectious disease like SARS, that's the best thing to do." Most of those who stayed home, though, quarantined themselves voluntarily: they were scared, and hid out at home, trying to weather the storm. In the rural areas, whole towns and villages closed themselves to outsiders, like European towns during a plague year.

The government enacted a sweeping series of measures the like of which have probably only been seen in the West during the Spanish flu epidemic after World War I. All movie theaters, discos, Internet bars, public libraries, and churches in the capital and also in Taiyuan, the capital of Shanxi province, were closed. On April 24, police sealed off one of the city's biggest hospitals, where there were at least 60 confirmed or suspected cases of SARS among the doctors and nurses. No one could enter the hospital, and the staff and patients at the hospital were forbidden to leave. A new thousand-bed "field hospital" was quickly set up on the outskirts of the city to deal with an expected overflow of patients. Beijing schools were closed, and 1.7 million students sent home. By the end of April the number of people in quarantine in the city had risen to at least 10,000. Some of the quarantined areas included whole villages in the suburbs of Beijing. In mid-May, by which time more than 5,000 people in China had been infected, the government announced that anyone who broke quarantine and infected others would be jailed or executed.

The government's response was matched by an equally dramatic popular response. "Within three days, two million people left Beijing," Bekedam said. "Pictures were taken in railway stations, bus stations, anywhere—it was massive."

The exodus took the infection to the provinces, and confirmed the WHO team's way of thinking: to remove the handle from the pump in a country such as China, it was crucial to monitor travel not only by air, but by any means. Just as the March WHO airline travel-screen advisory seems to have effectively prevented any new outbreaks, the April 30 Chinese domestic travel-screening order seems to have prevented a major transmission of SARS to the provinces, Bekedam said.

Like Hong Kong, Beijing became a city transformed. Dr. Anne Schuchat, a medical epidemiologist and internist, and Chief of the Respiratory Diseases Branch at the Centers for Disease Control and Prevention in Atlanta, saw the Chinese capital for the first time in May as part of the WHO team.

"If you've been there, you know this is an enormous extended urban landscape, [yet] it was empty. Coming in from the airport, our car was the only car on the road. I was staying in a hotel with others from the WHO team, and we were the only people in this 17-floor hotel, so there were probably 20 people staying in a hotel that had hundreds and hundreds of rooms. The restaurants were empty. They had closed most of the public venues, such as movie theaters. People who were bicycling were wearing masks, and anybody in any public setting was wearing a mask. Over the course of the time I was there, more and more public life resumed. Since it was my first trip there, I didn't realize how phenomenal the quiet and empty streets were. It was clear, towards the end, when there were traffic jams and cars and bikes on the streets, that was the normal Beijing.

"The medical task force was housed at a hotel, and this whole hotel had been taken over as the command center. It was a pretty efficient organization of people working 100 percent, 150 percent of their time, working there, sleeping there, eating there. If I arrived at the hotel at a certain point during the day, suddenly there would be all these official cars outside, and it would be the time when every hospital director from the designated SARS hospitals was there for the big meeting when they got their next instructions. In terms of the medical response, they had a very organized system: 'Okay, we were doing this, now we're going to do this instead, based on such-and-such.' It was a very efficient way to disseminate to the top leadership and take it back to their top institutions."

Her contact and colleague within the Beijing city authorities was Dr. Zhongan Zhu, a former director-general of the Beijing Health Bureau, who had been brought back from an academic position to coordinate the public health response between the Beijing government and the WHO.

"April, the third and fourth weeks, were a very terrible time, a very difficult time," he said over the phone, pausing often to find the right word. "The government issued information about the disease to the public. The public heard the information, but they didn't really know how to protect themselves against the disease. They were very scared."

Zhu quickly set up a series of task forces for different aspects of the operation, but everyone was finding they had to invent as they went along.

"We learned in medical school, public health school, all the classic epidemiological skills—set up a definition, gather as much data as possible, calculate... but those classical skills were not suitable for this kind of situation. We needed to make decisions on strategies for prevention and control very quickly, using very limited data, very limited knowledge and very limited time. The expert team had to submit a report and analysis of the situation, recommend strategies and what kinds of measures should be taken—in one or two days. Each day more than 100 probable new cases and another 100 suspected cases were being reported. There was so much work. It was really a crisis.

"We set up 16 SARS-designated hospitals for probable cases and 30 designated hospitals for suspected cases, and organized medical teams to work in these designated hospitals."

Zhu and his task forces set up an expert team in each hospital and fever clinic to examine suspected or probable cases to make a final decision. Clinics included medical observation rooms for unclear cases needing an overnight stay—a practice that other Chinese cities copied. They also set up special ICUs in SARS-designated hospitals for severe cases, with teams including respiratory disease specialists. They also recognized that because the patients were isolated in the hospitals, and because all the physicians and nurses wore serious protective equipment, these all created poor conditions for hospitalized patients, who got very depressed, especially as visitors and relatives were not allowed. "So what we did was to organize 16 psychological support teams, one for each designated hospital, to provide psychological care and support, which tremendously improved the outcome of the care."

They also worked on the aspect of the outbreak that was most novel and confusing for the general public: the new transparency.

"The public were worried because they didn't know a lot about the disease. The physicians and health bureau would not tell them a lot about the disease, but as we gradually learned more about the disease we told people what the real story was and to protect themselves, using the media. We used a hotline, the Internet, posters, radio, television and newspapers so the public wouldn't be as scared."

Curiously, amid all this turmoil things became in some respects calmer. The science writer Laurie Garrett reported that the official openness and the great volume of information now available meant that fewer people sent frantic rumors by cell phone text messaging.

" Last week such messages were frequent, offering such warnings as 'Do not go outside today. Authorities are moving hundreds of SARS patients and the air will not be safe.' Such text messaging has waned as the government has become more open about the epidemic."

China had to create modern public health out of the characteristic Chinese tangle of the ancient and modern. Zhu and his colleagues had to take a fragmented, superstitious, anxious, and suspicious public and forge a collective, purposeful body with a largely different set of beliefs and perceptions—and they had to do this in the middle of an epidemic.

Luckily, this is what the Chinese do well. It's a phenomenon that might be called pyramid-building: vast numbers of people are harnessed to carry out some huge public enterprise, and they do it in an orderly fashion almost overnight. It can be seen in physical form in the vast new cities of the Chinese Pacific coast. Now it had to be done in organizational form to create a public healthcare system capable of suppressing SARS.

Even as the broad-brush methods were beginning to stabilize the situation, Schuchat was working on some of the finer details.

For example: one of the diagnostic criteria for probable SARS was the combination of having pneumonia and recently coming from an "affected area." What do you do when the whole of Beijing has already been declared an affected area?

It was the old problem of signal-to-noise ratio: Beijing has 14 million people, among whom there were bound to be a sizeable number of common or garden variety pneumonias, and there was still no swift, accurate lab test for SARS. In Beijing, though, there were also new twists. Given the history of the past few months, health workers were on the highest level of alert for SARS, and could be forgiven for overdiagnosing. At the same time, both the press and health care forces coming in from outside were wary of official figures, suspecting more cover up. After the political crisis of mid-April, Schuchat said, "there was a feeling that 'We'd better talk about everything that's going on.' There was a perception on the part of health authorities and physicians that anything that might possibly be SARS, you'd better report." It wasn't just an accurate diagnosis that was important, but a credible one.

"The situation was challenging because we knew from what happened in Toronto or from the superspreader phenomenon that if you miss certain cases of SARS in terms of not setting up isolation around them, the disease could spread to a lot of other people. We had to have a very low threshold to consider someone potentially contagious."

Yet if they called every pneumonia a SARS, then the outbreak would seem far larger than it actually was, and accurate case numbers were vital: case numbers drove every aspect of the response, both local and international.

One of the main challenges facing the team of which Schuchat was a member was to try to work out what was going on with the patients who met the case definition of probable SARS (pneumonia with low white-blood-cell count, or with no improvement with antibiotics), but had no apparent link with any other infected person. Schuchat said, "The question was, 'Why do we have such a high proportion of unlinked cases?' One possibility was that there was so much transmission [going on] that you didn't know the person who infected you. You walked by them on the street, or you visited a hospital but it wasn't your uncle you were visiting in the hospital who infected you—it was somebody in the hallway, or the emergency room. Another possibility was that the district health investigators were just overwhelmed and didn't get all the data about recent contacts. Suddenly there were a hundred new cases being hospitalized every day, and they just couldn't keep up with it."

There was always the rogue possibility that the virus has found some new means of transmission, but in part the study was intended to rule out such a potential calamity, and to reduce such anxieties.

Their study asked a group of probable-SARS patients and a control group whether they had been into health care settings such as hospitals or fever clinics, whether they had been exposed to SARS patients in the community, whether they had been into live animal markets, to discover whether any of these factors correlated with having SARS. In a sense, epidemiology asks "What is going on?" It tries, by inference, to see the invisible.

"We did find that a substantial portion of cases had exposures to health care settings, either hospital visits (even though they didn't visit a person with SARS—they were in hospital for a clinical appointment, or accompanying a relative) or they were at one of these fever clinics, which were set up to try to triage, to separate the febrile from the non-febrile, and ideally to separate the SARS from the non-SARS" Schuchat added.

The fever clinics were an example of good public health gone wrong. They were set up in the name of early detection and isolation, and of taking the hospital out into the community, all of which are probably excellent intentions; but the infection control was so patchy that an investigation by Zhu shut down roughly half of the 100-plus clinics.

Schuchat said, "They really cut down transmission risk in fever clinics quite a bit, in terms of making sure that there was adequate training of personnel, that they had adequate supplies, and making sure that the physical set-up was such that you really could separate people coming in from each other."

Other reassuring news came in negative results. After the Amoy Gardens outbreak, rumors ran to Beijing that the virus had been transmitted by cats, rats, or cockroaches. "There were cartoons, there were announcements, there were threats," Schuchat said. "People were saying, 'Don't bring your pet into the elevator,' or 'Pets are going to be killed.' A lot of frenzy around that topic. So we asked about pets in our case-control study, not because we thought they were a risk factor." It turned out that pets, rats, and even roaches were innocent—of transmitting SARS, at least.

Finally, they found that a good number of the unlinked cases they studied didn't have antibody to the SARS coronavirus. So the mystery of the unlinked SARS cases was pretty well settled: it was still an epidemic, but even to know that an epidemic is business as usual can be very reassuring.

Another study addressed the issue of credibility. A number of cases seemed to be switching rapidly from "probable SARS" to "You can go home," and outsiders such as the WHO team were concerned in case this was a sign of a return to the no-outbreak-here mentality.

"The press was asking us constantly, 'Can we believe the numbers? Are the cases really going down?'" Schuchet and Dr. Weigong Zhou, a colleague from the CDC's Epidemic Intelligence Service reviewed cases from half-a-dozen hospitals, and "He found that they were mild illness that got [included in the broad SARS umbrella] temporarily, and under other circumstances most people would never have put this patient into the suspect category in the first place.

"The Beijing public health authorities wanted to be credible, but they were starting from a place where the press in particular, and WHO as well, were not open to trusting everything. They had to earn their credibility," Schuchat said.

By the time the outbreak was coming under control, what was straining credibility was the sheer scope and achievement of the Chinese response. Newcomers to Beijing, especially from the West, would say, "We don't understand why the cases are going away. We think they're faking the numbers." An outsider coming in at this stage of the outbreak might have no idea of how much work had been accomplished so quickly. Schuchat said, "The amount of training, the reassignment of vast numbers of health care staff, the construction of a new hospital....

"Here [in the United States] we would have probably spent quite a bit of time trying to figure out, 'Well, okay, it's a state of emergency, but who really has authority? Can we really order people to do this or that, whether it's the workers or the patients?' I think it would have been very challenging.

"They also had a pretty good system for getting education and communication information out at the neighborhood level. They were used to doing that for other reasons, so they knew how to do that pretty well. People would take their temperatures and the neighborhood monitor would get the logs. They had signs all over the place saying 'This is where your fever clinic is for this neighborhood. These are the signs and symptoms to watch for. This is how you should be cleaning and washing your hands and keeping your apartment clean. They really did that community-level door-to-door awareness that is probably more familiar to them" than it is in the United States.

"People were working incredibly hard. People in public health at the Beijing CDC—I mean, they were night and day in there, the place was just teeming with [activity], entering data, evaluating it, I can't remember how many phone lines they had set up... I was there later with someone from the New York City Health Department, which is a great health department, and she was just in awe of what the Beijing CDC had been able to do in response to [the outbreak] because it was just a massive human response. It was really an honor to work with them."

"Countries like China deal with multiple epidemics all the time," Mike Ryan, then Coordinator of GOARN, said with a combination of tactfulness and genuine sympathy. "Picking out those ones that are going to be a problem in three months' time is not an easy process. Once China recognized, openly, that they had a problem, once they engaged with the international community, their response was superb. I would challenge most countries in the world to be able to control SARS they way the Chinese did once they truly engaged in dealing with the problem transparently and aggressively."

SARS had been the lever that opened China's closed door. But by that time, matters were getting out of hand on an island just across a narrow but significant strait of ocean: Taiwan.

* * *

Infectious disease and politics are habitual bedfellows—a potent and dangerous combination, whether in the case of disease organisms being used for political ends, or nations playing politics during an outbreak and suffering as a result. Politics probably played a part to some degree every time the SARS virus crossed a border, like a patient suffering from inflammation and pain at every joint. In many cases this political element was probably not dangerous, consisting of little more than flag-waving and the customary expressions of blame and prejudice. In East Asia, though, where international cooperation was most important, the politics of SARS was fatal.

Taiwan's Center for Disease Control reported the first two suspected SARS cases on March 14: the two were a couple, of whom the man had recently traveled to Guangdong Province and Hong Kong. On March 26, a Taiwanese resident of Hong Kong's Amoy Gardens flew to Taiwan and took a train to Taichung to celebrate the traditional festival, Qing Ming. The man's brother became Taiwan's first SARS fatality, and a fellow passenger on the train was also infected.

Taiwan made two responses to these early cases, one medical, one political. While the cases were being competently treated, Taiwanese officials wrote a series of letters of protest to the WHO's Director-General, Dr. Brundtland. The complaint was familiar, futile, and frustrating, and the logic behind it ran like this. The WHO is a United Nations agency. In 1971, the United Nations decided that the People's Republic of China was, in essence, the authentic China, and the authentic China argued successfully that Taiwan was one of its provinces—something Taiwan vehemently denied, and continues to deny. This piece of political maneuvering meant that in the eyes of the UN, Taiwan ceased to exist as an independent nation. Because the WHO's charter allows it to deal only with the national governments of member nations, and then only by invitation, Taiwan found itself part of a global infectious disease outbreak but barred from calling on the WHO for help. The WHO could do nothing about the UN's decision, and was thus officially unable to respond.

Taiwan complained bitterly, with the strident tone of one used to being ignored:

"For many years, the People's Republic of China has been unreasonably opposed to Taiwan's joining the World Health

Organization. Recently, it has concealed information about a SARS outbreak in China, to result in a sudden global epidemic. The entire world is now under the threat of SARS, and global economy may thus be seriously affected adversely. It is obvious that China is interfering health matters with politics. Such interference will not only bring about harm to its own people, but is also hazardous to the world."

"China has told the world they are taking care of us," said Taiwan's Premier Yu Shyi-kun. "It's a shameless lie."

In addition to petitioning the WHO, Taiwan petitioned the health minister of every WHO member state to support Taiwan's bid to become an observer at the World Health Congress, a position that would give the island nation at least affiliate status within the WHO.

Health Minister Twu Shing-jer also appealed for assistance to the U.S. Department of Health and Human Services and the Centers for Disease Control and Prevention, and also to the WHO.

Political help may not have been forthcoming, but medical help was. Experts from the U.S. Centers for Disease Control and Prevention flew to Taiwan early in the outbreak, followed (when China consented) by an official WHO team on May 3, though they were officially forbidden to talk to Taiwanese health officials. Still, one senior Taiwanese physician reported that there was no shortage of outside expertise available, even if some of it was delivered, as he put it, "under the table."

At first, despite Taiwan's political-outsider status, the epidemic on the island seemed to be mild. Between early March and April 20 (officially, at least) most of the fewer than thirty30 SARS cases were travel-related, and there were as yet no fatalities.

This good news, however, became political currency. As late as April 21, Taiwan's health officials were still hailing their "success" in preventing SARS at an international conference in Taipei, comparing their own situation favorably with those in China and Hong Kong, and claiming that it represented the superiority of Taiwan's "liberal democratic ideals" over mainland China's protracted cover-up of the disease.

The government was playing on its own stage, the medical profession had an outbreak to contend with.

"The SARS outbreak in Taiwan had two phases," said Dr Chen Pei-Jer, a molecular virologist at the National Taiwan University. Chen was asked to be part of a team of virologists, immunologists, and epidemiologists to study SARS, initially in the university hospital (the

National Taiwan University Hospital) and then in other hospitals on the island. They sequenced the virus and then examined its genetic structure, ultimately sequencing and doing molecular analysis on 12 strains of the virus.

"The first phase was in early March until the middle of April," Chen said. "The first case was treated at our university hospital. At that time we didn't know what kind of infectious agent was causing the disease so we just took universal precautions and treated it as a new emerging infectious disease. During that time, every day we had only two or three cases, and they were all imported, either from China or from Hong Kong or by way of other countries. The government or the health authorities caught them in time. Sporadic cases can be contained very easily.

"Later, though, there was a big problem. In one hospital, in the municipal hospital in Taipei, there was an unrecognized case. And that case spread and caused an outbreak all over the entire island. This had nothing to do with China. The failure was due to the local government, or even the local health authorities, for example in Taipei City. They did not do their job well enough. China did have their responsibility: they really were a bit late to take precautions. But other countries also had the same problem. This is just my view, but I cannot scold China too much."

The official version of what happened next is that Taiwan's President Chen Shui-bian received a phone call on April 22 from a friend, a local health care official, warning him that Ho Ping Municipal Hospital in Taipei was covering up an outbreak of SARS among its patients and medical staff. He dispatched a team of investigators from Taiwan's CDC, and sure enough, a new cluster of seven infections was found, starting a chain of transmission that led to 116 probable cases and 10 deaths in two weeks, 264 cases and 34 deaths by mid-May, and 680 cases and 81 deaths in less than a month. Two months after the initial WHO alert, Taiwan had the third-worst SARS epidemic in the world, and its health care system came close to collapse.

Ho Ping Municipal Hospital was shut down on April 24 when the situation spiraled out of control and 200 patients and 900 staff were compulsorily quarantined.

The outbreak spread so rapidly and widely through the health care system that at least nine major hospitals were either fully or partly shut down, and more than 150 doctors and nurses refused to return to work because they were so angry at the apparent lack of overall management of the outbreak and scared for their lives because of poor infection control.

One doctor spoke to the Western press of the situation in late April, when hundreds of staff, patients, and visitors were locked inside together for days, unsure of who was sick, short of masks and gowns, and with no one really in charge.

"That was a violation of human rights," he said.

The government, in turn, threatened to revoke the licenses of doctors and nurses who refused to return to the front-an approach that did little to calm fears among hospital workers. Although only a small percentage had walked out, those who remained had good reason to be scared, says Tseng Jean-lie, chairman of the National Union of Nurses Association. "In some of the hospitals, medical staff are supplied with only two masks a week," says Tseng. "They should be getting a new one every four hours. It's not good enough."

The hazardous conditions led to further confrontations when nurses protested their low pay—one-tenth of what doctors earn, according to the Taipei City Nurses Association.

"A starting nurse makes $570 to $860 a month," reported the *New York Times*, "while Taiwan's minimum wage is $430. Hospitals are now offering up to $143 a day in 'danger pay' for working on SARS wards, but [the Nurses Association] said it was unfairly distributed. Doctors get much more even though they spend less time with patients. SARS nurses are virtually shut into isolation wards for eight hours at a stretch in masks, face shields, and triple gowns that make it hard to use bathrooms and all but impossible to eat safely."

In an effort to stem the defections, the government offered a range of compensation for any professional infected with SARS while caring for SARS patients: $350,000 Taiwan dollars (TWD) (a little over $10,000 U.S.), rising to $10 million TWD for anyone who died or was left handicapped, plus educational expenses for surviving children.

These were not the only unusual steps officials took to try to contain the epidemic. The government offered T$2,500 (US$72) cash rewards for informants who tipped off health authorities on new SARS infections. "People who suspect their family members, close friends, or neighbors may be infected with SARS can report them to local health authorities," a Department of Health official said. Taipei Mayor Ma Ying-jeou introduced a new and almost panoramically broad case definition by proposing an automatic three-day quarantine for anyone with a fever. The Department of Health banned drugstores from selling anti-fever pills to force possible SARS sufferers to go to see doctors, and Taipei's roads were gridlocked when a government order that all subway and train passengers should wear masks convinced many commuters that public transport was unsafe.

These measures led to more disagreement between the political and medical professions.

"Health officials have misled people with their extreme moves," said Ruey Lin, an epidemiology expert at National Taiwan University's Public Health Department. "They need to give proper information so people know communal infection risk is very low."

In the hospitals, unfortunately, the infection risk was very high. If the world needed Toronto to illustrate the devastating effects of missing a single undiagnosed patient, perhaps Taiwan's value was to illustrate the importance of inter-hospital tracking. On April 26, a female patient from Taipei was transferred from the emergency department of Kaohsiung Chang Gung Memorial Hospital to Ward X for treatment. Nobody, apparently, asked about her history of contacts.

Two days later she declined to the point of needing emergency intubation, in the course of which she vomited on a nurse and two doctors. It wasn't until two days later that the hospital learned that she had previously been seen at the Jenchi Hospital, where a SARS infection was raging. The hospital put 10 medical and nursing staff who had had contact with her in the E.R. and 37 who had seen her between April 26 and 30 into a quarantine ward. The nurse and one of the doctors who had intubated her fell sick within days; two weeks later the doctor died.

Ward X became an infection epicenter: nine medical and nursing staff, 17 patients and 18 family members became infected, and even two undertakers who had handled the bodies of SARS patients fell sick.

The Taiwan outbreak also featured what must be one of the unluckiest instances of transmission. When the Ho Ping index case was X-rayed, and as soon as the X-rays revealed possible SARS, the X-ray room was disinfected. Somehow, though, the patient's gown was overlooked. Some time later a hospital laundry worker came along and collected the gown for laundering. When he fell sick, he was treated for salmonella infection, so the health care staff around him didn't wear full protective equipment, and more infections resulted.

Dark rumors surfaced about the hospitals. Nurses interviewed by Time said that SARS-like symptoms had been seen in patients in Ho Ping since April 9, that the criteria for diagnosing SARS were unclear, that infection control equipment had been grossly inadequate, and that they had been ordered to reclassify all probable SARS cases as "pneumonia" cases and tell families that there was no SARS in Taiwan—a recipe for disaster already demonstrated by Taiwan's rival, China. The hospital was fined $75,000 for failing to report cases sooner.

Twu Shiing-jer, Minister of Health, and Chen Tzay-jinn, director of the CDC, resigned. The director of Ho Ping Hospital was dismissed and charged with negligence, yet many felt that these were scapegoats for wider and more systemic problems.

At the height of the outbreak, on May 19, Beijing blocked Taiwan's appeal to the WHO World Health Assembly to join the WHO as an observer, arguing that Taiwan was not a UN member state and that Taiwan could always receive WHO assistance through mainland China.

Immediately after this frustrating and humiliating setback for Taiwan, China offered to send a substantial cargo of medical supplies, including 200,000 protective gowns, 100,000 N95 face masks and five ambulances, across the strait to Taiwan. The Taiwanese government was caught in a political trap: if it accepted the offer, it would implicitly be demonstrating its reliance on China and weakening its bid to be an independent member of the WHO and the UN. On the other hand, if it refused the offer it would seem to be playing politics at the expense of its own people. In the end, independence won out, and the aid was turned down.

The official Chinese news agency, Xinhua, retaliated in no uncertain terms, saying that, thanks to "the selfish, personal political interests of 'pro-independence' separatists, the health of the Taiwanese people has been ignored."

It's hard to say for sure how the politics of the outbreak affected the ultimate outcome of the epidemic, but Taiwan was the last country to be removed, on July 5th, from the WHO's list of areas still infected by the virus.

A year later, the following editorial could still be read on Taiwan's Center for Disease Control website:

"China is a country where politics always interferes with health matters. In China, not only disease information is not transparent, epidemics are often left alone without proper management. Such incompetence in disease control brings harm to the health of its own people, and that of the world population as well. The international community should realize by now, from the ways China and Taiwan handle the SARS outbreaks, which one of them is fulfilling its responsibilities as a member of the global community, and which one is endangering the health of the peoples of the world."

Chapter 18.
It Wasn't Magic Any More

If the outbreak began like a series of global fireworks, rocketing out of southern China and exploding in quick succession all over the globe, it ended less dramatically and less coherently, fizzling out in one place while it still burned in another.

In individual countries, the end of the epidemic was marked by a steady diminution of novelty and alarm: the unknown was becoming known. The horrifying assault on hospitals, the inexplicable leaps that took down healthy people by the handful or even the dozen were now, as the medical terminology says, "well understood," even if specific questions remained, and still remain today. The virus had lost its aura: it was now just a disease.

Dr. Aileen Plant, working in Hanoi, felt this shift. "It was about the middle of April before I thought, 'Yeah, I think it's going to be okay. We still had to wait a bit longer until we got the all clear, but we felt that things were under control and we felt that it wasn't magic anymore. It was a virus. We knew how it was going to behave, and if we could just get people quickly and get them isolated once they had symptoms, they wouldn't infect anymore people. And then all we had to do was find all their contacts and make sure they didn't get symptoms, or if they did get symptoms, they were in turn isolated. Once you start to get to that stage where you think, 'This is just a virus. It's a nuisance. It seems to spread reasonably easily, but it is actually controllable,' then I started to feel a bit happier."

The WHO declared SARS contained in Viet Nam on April 28, 2003; it was the first country to successfully contain an outbreak of any size.

What turned the corner for Viet Nam, as it would do for every country, was successful containment, which for practical purposes consisted of infection control and contact tracing. As early as April 12, evidence came in that new infection control procedures at the Prince of Wales Hospital had dramatically reduced infection rates among hospital staff: doctors, from 75 percent to 5 percent; nurses from 79 percent to 6 percent; other staff from 42 percent to 4 percent; and the infection risk to the families of health care staff had dropped to zero.

It wasn't the beginning of the end but, in Winston Churchill's phrase, it might have been the end of the beginning.

Other institutions adopted different procedures at different times, but by the end of April the message was clear: after an initial burst of imported cases and infections within families or in the community, the bulk of the cases—as many as 90 percent—would be hospital-acquired infections, and in the end it was routine hygiene that defeated SARS. A very different set of routines, to be sure, involving new equipment, new vigilance, new rigor, but nothing that any hospital in the world could not adopt.

All the same, someone was needed to provide evidence of how disastrous it was to miss a single diagnosis of SARS, and it was Toronto's misfortune to provide this salutary lesson.

As was generally the case, it wasn't clear for some time how what was called Phase Two started. The first sign of danger was in late May when a patient in a rehab center after a double-lung transplant became ill. A bronchoscopy was performed, bringing back bad news: SARS coronavirus. Contact tracing took investigators back up the chain to North York General Hospital.

"Toronto Public Health sent a team in expecting to find maybe one case," Bonnie Henry, Associate Medical Officer of Health, said glumly. "By the end of the day they found at least a dozen." Many could be identified only retrospectively; two had already died. Four hospitals were immediately declared to be Category Three: "hospital has someone with SARS and there has already been probable transmission within that hospital."

Barbara Yaffe, the Acting Medical Officer of Health who had announced the initial outbreak, now had to go back out and announce what is universally referred to as Phase Two. At the beginning of the original outbreak, nobody knew what they were getting into, and there was a certain sense of frantic adventure. By now everyone was burned and scarred, and it was all too clear what the return of the virus meant. "I felt sick," Yaffe said. "I knew the panic that would potentially ensue. But there was no choice. I had to do it, and I had to do it right away."

Yaffe had had an exceptionally tough time during the outbreak. Her mother fell ill with heart trouble right before Phase One, and was admitted to a hospital. Then SARS struck, and the hospital was closed to visitors. Her mother, old, sick, confused, and failing quickly, didn't understand what was happening. "You don't love me," she told her daughter over the phone. "You're not coming to see me." When it became clear that her mother wasn't going to get better, Yaffe tried to get her released to come home to die, but community home care and other services refused to transport anyone out of a hospital for fear of broadcasting the virus. Eventually Yaffe got her mother home, and she died during the outbreak.

By May 23, health officials announced that Phase Two consisted of at least 25 suspected and probable cases at two Toronto hospitals, and that two recent deaths might have been caused by SARS. At least 500 people were put in quarantine.

Karietha Cooke, working as a liaison in the hospitals, had noticed a change in the human dynamics around her during Phase One. The infection control practitioners began to treat her as an equal, a colleague. Hospital staff and public health staff, physicians and social workers—"There was an understanding that everyone was in it for the public good."

This spirit of camaraderie was wrecked by the onset of Phase Two. "People were already burned out. Everyone had been working seven days a week, up to 16 hours a day. Forget about seeing your family."

In some respects, Cooke said, the administration of Phase Two was handled much better, and the outbreak was controlled more quickly. She was transferred to Scarborough General, where a command center had been set up in the boardroom, staffed with infection control practitioners, public health staff, epidemiologists, physicians, risk management coordinators, the hospital administrators—everyone who needed to work together.

By now, though, everyone was running on fumes. "People were very irritable. There was stress and anxiety almost to the point of nervous breakdown," Cooke said.

The public's patience for quarantine had also worn very thin. Bonnie Henry had noticed a parabola of resistance. "It's very difficult to do contact tracing. People forget. They don't want to identify people. They especially don't want to identify their friends. People were angry when we called, especially early on. And then in Phase Two it went back to anger and frustration again."

The consensus is that, with the lessons learned already, Phase Two was brought under control far more quickly, and on July 2, the WHO removed Toronto from its list of SARS-affected cities, no new infections having been reported for 20 days, twice the incubation period.

This was hardly the end of SARS in the province, though: two days later the funeral was held for Nelia Laroza, the first Canadian health care worker to die from SARS, who had passed away at the end of June. On July 20, a second nurse died of SARS, having battled the virus since the first outbreak. On August 11, the last private citizen of Toronto died of SARS, and two days later Dr. Nestor Yanga becomes the first North American doctor to die of SARS, which he had contracted while treating a SARS patient more than four months previously.

It would be misleading to end an account of the outbreak on such a note, though. What emerged time and again as people spoke about their experiences in Toronto (and elsewhere) and their story drew toward a close was a sense that something terrible and exhausting had happened, but something remarkable had taken place too, and this was often the last thing people spoke about.

In Geri Nephew's case it was the fact that, even though the beginning of Phase Two was busier than any time except the very start of Phase One, there was an influx of help—colleagues who came in response to personal invitations that amounted to begging. New staff, mostly public health nurses and public health investigators, came in from elsewhere in the province. Three from Hamilton. Ten from London. People from Grey-Bruce and Huron. "It was so great to see new faces. That was one of the best things that happened," Nephew said. Health Canada sent physicians and epidemiologists from across the country. An amazing epidemiologist came from National Defense, another from Vancouver, and another from one of the shelters in Toronto.

By the end of each country's outbreak, whatever the date, everyone involved was exhausted, yet time and again people told me that a remarkable change had taken place. SARS, like many an ordeal, had brought people together, at every level from the local to the global, in a common struggle. In doing so, it had not only given people a new appreciation for each other's efforts, it had also given them a brief preview of how new collaborative medical and social practices might be made permanent.

Clinicians and researchers, often in their own separate professional universes, had worked together. Hospital staff had started listening to their infection-control officers, and working more actively with local public health officials. People who normally ignored each other in the elevator now exchanged greetings and news, and countries that had ignored each other now exchanged data and emails. Health care workers took leave of their usual jobs, sometimes without pay, and went to a different town, or province, or country to help out.

* * *

What of those countries that didn't have substantial outbreaks? (See Table 1.)

Table 1.

Country	Cumulative No. of Case(s)	No. of Deaths	Case Fatality Ratio (%)
Australia	6	0	0
Canada	251	43	17
China	5327	349	7
France	7	1	14
Germany	9	0	0
Hong Kong	1755	299	17
India	3	0	0
Indonesia	2	0	0
Italy	4	0	0
Kuwait	1	0	0
Macao	1	0	0
Malaysia	5	2	40
Mongolia	9	0	0
New Zealand	1	0	0
Philippines	14	2	14
Republic of Ireland	1	0	0
Republic of Korea	3	0	0
Romania	1	0	0
Russian Federation	1	0	0
Singapore	238	33	14
South Africa	1	1	100
Spain	1	0	0
Sweden	5	0	0
Switzerland	1	0	0
Taiwan	346	37	11
Thailand	9	2	22
United Kingdom	4	0	0
United States*	29	0	9
Viet Nam	63	5	8
Total	8,098	774	9.6

(WHO, current as of 10/2003)
**According to the CDC in mid-2004, the United States had 161 possible SARS cases, with 134 of them suspect, 19 probable, and 8 laboratory confirmed. The latter two categories add up to 27.*

The difference between countries that had significant outbreaks and those that didn't was largely a matter of alertness, timing, caution, and luck.

In the United States, as in many countries, the first hints turned up in the ProMED discussions of February 10, 2003, and from then on the Centers for Disease Control and Prevention (CDC) in Atlanta was watching South China very closely for signs of pandemic influenza. But in the United States, a secondary possibility needed to be considered: the threat of bioterrorism.

"You can imagine what we thought when we heard the room 911 story," said Dr. Jim Hughes, Director of the National Center for Infectious Disease (NCID) at the CDC. "I can guarantee you that law enforcement and intelligence were very interested—as they should be." Luckily, it was clear from early in the outbreak that natural causes were at work

The CDC was already primed to react, thanks in particular to two previous events: a 1993 hantavirus outbreak in the southwest, which produced its own version of a severe acute respiratory syndrome, and the anthrax letters of October 2001. The latter in particular had brought an awareness in the United States that a national security threat might well overlap in almost every respect with a public health threat, and sent a cascade of funding toward public health, traditionally a poor cousin in the U.S. health care system.

By a remarkable piece of synchrony, the CDC's new Emergency Operations Center, which had been opened less than a week earlier, was a well-equipped new war room for emergencies that might include acts of bioterrorism or outbreaks of infectious disease. The CDC's director, Dr. Julie Gerberding, activated it on March 14, 2003, when the first SARS alerts came out of Toronto. "We moved in on March 15," Hughes said, "and we were in there for 135 days."

One of the lessons of the anthrax alert was that CDC needed to vastly improve communications, so the Emergency Communications System was set up to link a series of constituencies: clinical, public health, policy and the general public, setting up hotlines, using the Internet, and establishing a feedback loop to find out how well the message was being heard.

On March 17, 2003, shortly after the emergency response started, national surveillance for SARS in the United States began. This was facilitated by the CDC's Epidemic Information Exchange (Epi-X), a secure public health communications network. Two interesting aspects of this process were that even in such an outbreak, the reporting remained "passive," i.e., rather than going out and identifying cases, the public health people relied on their medical colleagues to report potential cases. The other aspect was reminiscent of other regions as well, in that much of the recording and reporting from hospitals to state-level agencies to the CDC took place on paper (or via telephone) rather than electronically. At the CDC, the epidemiologic data were eventually compiled in electronic form and run against laboratory data.

As it turned out, some of the more effective tools were travel advisory notices handed out to air passengers returning from SARS-affected regions, which recommended they contact their physician if they suffered from any of the given list of symptoms. Many, perhaps most referrals came from this source.

Early information came in from a lab in Bangkok, Thailand, staffed with three CDC employees who worked with Dr. Carlo Urbani. Atlanta heard very quickly how communicable the disease was, and how dangerous. Word went out rapidly to clinical and infection-control practitioners. The first SARS Health Alert notices went out March 16, 2003, for passengers arriving at Chicago, Los Angeles, New York, and San Francisco airports inbound from Hong Kong.

The CDC was also helped by having small existing quarantine offices and personnel at eight major international airports in the United States who were accustomed to dealing with incoming problems on airplanes. The system is presently being increased in coverage, as a result of SARS and bioterrorism concerns, to as many as 25 airports.

Even so, there were holes in the defense. One suspect case flew back from Asia to southern California and, despite feeling ill, wanted to continue the journey home by train. "We really didn't want that to happen," Hughes said, but there was initially nothing that could be done legally to stop the passenger. Fortunately, the patient felt sufficiently sick to get off the train and check into a hospital; even more fortunately, the cause was not SARS. Even so, cases like this prompted the CDC and the Department of Health and Human Services to ask the President to sign an executive order including SARS on the list of quarantinable diseases.

Just as the WHO had its network of influenza laboratories and its virtual network of labs working to identify and sequence the SARS coronavirus (SARS-CoV), the CDC had its own Laboratory Response Network of more than a 100 labs in the United States that collaborated on the hunt for the SARS virus. This network, too, was a response to the anthrax scare, and was put in place for the familiar combination of bioterrorism and infectious disease purposes.

Over the course of the outbreak, CDC mobilized more than 850 people to work on SARS (see Table 2). More than 90 were sent abroad in various capacities. According to the CDC, the United States ended up with 161 possible cases, with 134 of them suspect, 19 probable, and 8 laboratory confirmed. Two of the latter were a family pair who stayed at the Metropole.

Table 2.

Country	No. of Staff Deployed	No. of Days Deployed
Taiwan	30	696
China	17	498
Vietnam	10	226
Singapore	5	137
Philippines	4	98
Hong Kong	6	88
Thailand	4	60
Canada/Ottawa	5	57
Canada/Toronto	4	46
Switzerland	4	33
Cambodia	1	15
Laos	2	5

Total staff deployed: 92 Total days deployed: 1,959

"We were on this quickly," Hughes said, "and the front-line [clinical] people were onto it quickly, but frankly we could have had a Toronto experience. If we had had a superspreader on March 14, I can guarantee you we would have had a problem."

The SARS experience has not left him feeling reassured about the prospect of another global pandemic, such as influenza.

"The next 'flu pandemic will happen. And our response won't work nearly as well as it did with SARS", warned Hughes. Patients with SARS didn't become infectious until they were already showing symptoms of the disease; flu transmission takes place before or as symptoms appear, so isolation and quarantine won't work nearly as well.

[Editor's Note: The U.S. pandemic influenza plan, 10 years in the making, was released for public discussion on August 25, 2004.]

* * *

In general, the first wave of exported virus broke across the world largely irrespective of the quality of local health care and surveillance systems; in Toronto, several infections had already taken place even before the first SARS patient saw a doctor. From then on, it was a question of whether individual physicians or hospital staff had paid attention to the alert and how cautious they were in their handling of the patient, whether high-risk procedures such as emergency intubation were needed, how good the infection-control practices were, how sick the patient was when he or she arrived in a medical setting, plus the strange capriciousness of the virus—many of which were factors beyond anyone's reasonable control.

A more significant factor was the amount of international travel between the destinations. It has often been said that the world was lucky that SARS didn't strike the world's poorest nations, but the world's poorest nations, with the exception of some of the western Pacific nations, were less likely to have travelers visiting them from South China.

Once the virus had been recognized and the WHO alert had gone out—and here the speed of the WHO response was critical—nations were far better prepared to recognize and deal with incoming cases. So Japan, for example, despite being in the Western Pacific, the SARS hot zone, had several cases but no outbreak. In fact, one of the fascinating facts about the epidemic is that with the possible exception of Taiwan, there were no new outbreaks following the WHO warning. There were existing outbreaks that bubbled up or renewed themselves, and there were new imported individual cases, but the original means of transmission, the one that everyone had been fearing—that aircraft would criss-cross the world, infecting country after country and setting off nationwide outbreaks—did not happen.

The SARS virus started regardless of the host country's abilities-only after initial spread had occurred was the quality of response a factor. Perhaps the salient observation here is Mike Ryan's comment: Everyone gets it wrong at first. After that, it's a question of how quickly you recover.

Chapter 19.

Aftershocks

After the official end of the outbreak, only the foolhardy were throwing away their masks and announcing a return to life as usual. The source of the original outbreak in Guangdong had not been found, so there was always the possibility that it would flare up again, and given that the SARS virus turned out to be a coronavirus, and cold viruses are coronaviruses, and colds tend to be seasonal, and the outbreak had taken off in flu season, nobody would have been surprised if SARS returned in East Asia with the return of winter at the end of 2003.

As things turned out, the virus continued to keep humankind guessing. The cold-and-flu season brought no SARS revival, but in the nine months after July 5 at least 10 new cases of SARS emerged, one fatal, all raising questions.

Less than two months after the WHO declared the outbreak officially contained, a 27-year-old post-doctoral student working on insect-born pathogens in Singapore's Environmental Health Institute (EHI) was infected with the virus. The details of the accident were not released, but the researcher was apparently working with the SARS, West Nile, and dengue fever viruses, and the West Nile sample apparently became contaminated with SARS. Investigators pointed out that the EHI was a lower biosafety level lab that had been pressed into service during the outbreak and was still being used for hazardous research.

"Inappropriate laboratory standards and a cross-contamination of West Nile virus samples with SARS coronavirus in the laboratory led to the infection of the doctoral student," the WHO investigating committee reported. Nobody else, apparently, was infected, and the post-doc recovered.

The Singapore incident was still fresh in the public mind in mid-December when the health minister of Taiwan announced that another medical researcher, testing various medicines on the SARS virus in a military hospital, had become infected on December 6.

A 44-year-old researcher, identified only as Lieutenant Colonel Chan, had been screening antiviral drugs for effectiveness against the SARS coronavirus at the National Defense University in Taipei. According to the investigating committee, the SARS virus samples were handled within a closed cabinet using attached gloves, in accordance with WHO recommendations for a BSL-4 lab. A transporting chamber that could be securely attached to the cabinet was used to transfer waste materials to an autoclave for sterilization. Chan noticed that some liquid waste had spilled into the chamber. Unable to reach the material through the attached gloves, he sprayed the area with alcohol and waited 10 minutes. Thinking it had been disinfected, Chan then opened the transporting chamber door to finish cleaning up—an act that probably exposed him to the virus.

Following the now familiar SARS pattern, the researcher caught a plane on December 7, attended a conference in Singapore and then flew back to Taiwan on December 10, by which time he had begun to develop fever symptoms. He was admitted to a hospital on December 16, and SARS was diagnosed the next day. Contact tracing was carried out at once in both countries; Singapore quarantined 70 people who had been in close contact with the researcher.

Over the next few days, however, it became clear that only sheer luck, and the usual capriciousness of the virus, prevented a far more serious breach. When the researcher developed symptoms on December 10, he spent the night at his work dormitory, then put on a mask and had his wife drive him to a clinic in suburban Taipei. He then waited another five days before going to a hospital. Moreover, he had traveled to and from Singapore with two colleagues who had since flown to the United States. Amazingly, none of these contacts seem to have developed SARS.

As if to underline how little had been learned from these accidents, and how dangerous the SARS virus is, the most serious lab accident to date took place in China's most prestigious SARS research lab, in the Beijing Center for Disease Control, in spring 2004. A 26-year-old graduate student, Ms. Song, somehow contracted SARS while working in the lab, before taking thc train south to her home in Anhui Province on March 23. Two days later, she developed a fever; on March 29 she returned to Beijing, again by train. She was treated for viral pneumonia in both Beijing and Anhui, but by April 6 her mother, who had cared for her at home and traveled by train with her, and a nurse in a hospital where Song had been treated, had become infected. Her mother died of an undiagnosed respiratory infection that only afterwards was considered as possible SARS, despite the daughter's connection with the lab. By April 25, the Chinese government had sealed off the lab, had identified at least 300 contacts, and found a total of six possible SARS cases, all traceable to Ms. Song.

These accidents were a vivid demonstration that the virus could not be underestimated or forgotten. It might be in captivity, but it had by no means been domesticated. Many laboratories around the world, according to the *New York Times*, have stored thousands of SARS specimens in freezers, ready to be thawed as needed. "In China we're doing all that is possible," said Dr. Henk Bekedam, "but we still can't be sure that all the specimens are being kept in the right places and are being handled in the right ways."

The incident was also a disturbing echo of an earlier lab accident. Months after smallpox had been eradicated, a notorious accident occurred in 1979, when the virus escaped from a laboratory at the University of Birmingham in England. It infected two people, one fatally, and the head of the laboratory committed suicide.

We now know that smallpox was also being kept elsewhere and developed in bioweapons programs.

The concept of eradication, then, is a misnomer. An "eradicated" virus, spore, bacillus, or parasite is unlikely to be completely absent from the earth. Instead, it is in containment, where it may face three possible forms of emergence and activity: medical research, accident, or bioweapon. Two of the three are profoundly unpleasant outcomes; the onus on both lab safety and lab supervision is therefore enormous, and the SARS lab incidents didn't give much cause for confidence on either score.

* * *

The other three cases all occurred in China, and to understand them, and a great deal of the late SARS activity in China, we need to go back to May 23, 2003, when a joint research project by teams from both Hong Kong and Shenzhen, the major Chinese city immediately across the border from Hong Kong, introduced the world to the potential dangers of the civet cat.

The researchers, including Dr. K-Y Yuen of the University of Hong Kong, were following up on the observation, early in the Guangdong phase of the epidemic, that a high proportion of those initially infected had connections to the business of raising, selling, butchering, or cooking food—specifically, food from the live wild-animal markets of South China.

Chinese tradition holds that the careful selection of food is extremely important for health. Ideally, meat should be bought while still alive, then butchered and eaten fresh—wise advice in the days before refrigeration, when contamination of dead meat was common and often lethal. In particular, one tradition held that when the weather started to turn cold during late autumn and early winter, it was important to eat wild animals— the theory presumably being that the qualities that enable wildlife to endure the harsh weather are likely to be most useful to humans, too, at that time of year. These traditions were very much alive in Guangdong, where residents had acquired a taste for certain wild animals in particular.

A new virus has to come from somewhere, and the fact that the infection had initially been so common among food-handlers suggested that SARS was zoonotic—that is, it had jumped the species barrier from an animal, possibly one in the live markets.

Sure enough: Dr. Yuen said, "The study detected several coronaviruses closely related genetically to the SARS coronavirus in two of the animal species tested (masked palm civet and raccoon dog). The study also found that one additional species (the Chinese ferret badger) elicited antibodies against the SARS-CoV. These and other wild animals are traditionally considered delicacies and are sold for human consumption in markets throughout southern China."

"In the past month," Yuen told reporters," we have been able to do a lot of work on sampling the fecal material of the wild animals, and from a special type of civet, civet cat, we are able to isolate the coronavirus. And this coronavirus on genomic analysis was found to be very, very similar to the coronavirus causing SARS in humans."

All six of the civets—not a kind of cat at all, but a relative of the mongoose—in the study were found to harbor a virus virtually identical to what science now officially calls SARS-CoV, or the SARS coronavirus. Moreover, blood samples from animal and vegetable traders in the market found that 40 percent of the animal traders, 20 percent of the animal butchers, and 5 percent of the vegetable traders had traces of SARS, although none reported SARS symptoms over the last six months.

Other studies found SARS also in macaques, fruit bats, snakes, and wild pigs, and 66 out of 508 animal handlers tested at several Guangdong markets had antibodies against the SARS virus—in other words, they had been exposed to it at some point.

"At present, no evidence exists to suggest that these wild animal species play a significant role in the epidemiology of SARS outbreaks," the study concluded cautiously. "However, it cannot be ruled out that these animals might have been a source of human infection."

At once, two sides developed. On one side was the substantial portion of Guangdong residents who liked wild-animal meat, including those who made a living selling it, who argued with some justification that there was no proof of a single person catching SARS from a wild animal. The civet could have passed the virus to another animal that passed it to humans, or some third-party animal might have passed the virus to the civet, which passed it to humans. By now it was clear that numerous other species, ranging from rats to domestic cats, could carry the SARS virus, and no one yet knew how or even if any of these species could transmit the virus to humans—or whether these animals were infected by humans rather than the other way round.

On the other side was an increasingly frustrated medical establishment—especially outside China—that had just survived a major global epidemic and now at last had a clue, no matter how circumstantial, as to where it might all have started.

Trapped between these constituencies was the Guangdong provincial government—and, to some extent, the WHO, which was now working closely and extensively with medical authorities in China to find reasonable and evidence-based solutions in an increasingly difficult situation.

In late May, Guangdong officials were reported to be showing a sudden interest in protecting endangered animals, the same species that had been sold in the marketplace for decades. Meanwhile, thousands of markets, restaurants, and kitchens throughout Guangdong were raided, shut down, and hosed clean in a desperate attempt to wash away the virus.

The Guangdong authorities, according to Yuen, tried to adopt a middle-ground policy by banning sales of the SARS-implicated animals, then lifted the ban in August, after several months had passed with no cases of SARS—a move that left the WHO, in Bekedam's words, "not amused."

As if in response, starting in mid-December 2003, four cases emerged in quick succession, all in the province of Guangdong: a 32-year-old television producer, a 20-year-old waitress working in a Guangzhou restaurant with civet on the menu, a 35-year-old businessman, and a 40-year old director of a hospital and practicing physician from Guangzhou.

The television producer protested that he had never even seen civet cats, let alone eaten them, but the Chinese authorities now, according to Yuen, decided they had to take the threat seriously—a move that the WHO, which had been working closely with Beijing and Guangdong to investigate both the cases and the possible animal origins of SARS, welcomed. "WHO today welcomed a decision by the Chinese authorities to try and minimize contact between humans and the animals thought to be carrying the SARS virus," announced a WHO press release.

"WHO has long maintained that animals could be reservoirs for the SARS CoV, and hence a source of infection," said Dr Hitoshi Oshitani, who leads WHO's response to SARS in the Western Pacific Region. "WHO has repeatedly called for more research to identify which animals are capable of carrying and transmitting the virus to humans, and, very importantly, under what circumstances the virus is able to transmit from animals to humans.",

What the WHO (and the central government in Beijing) meant by "minimizing contact" and "more research" may not have been exactly what the Guangdong authorities had in mind. Over several days in early January an estimated 10,000 civets were electrocuted, incinerated, drowned in disinfectant, or "liquefied in pressurized pots."

Oshitani cautioned that if wild animals were to be slaughtered, the people carrying out the cull should be protected from infection. "The cull should be done cautiously," he said.

Oshitani's warning was clearly not passed on to those in the field.

"A crowd gathered to watch men in white and blue jumpsuits throw bags of the animals into a truck," reported the Associated Press. "When one civet leapt out, a worker grabbed it by the neck with heavy tongs while another hit it over the head with a metal rod. Police were on hand to push onlookers back. Afterward, workers wearing goggles and rubber boots sprayed chemical disinfectant around the stall."

Not only were the authorities killing off the most valuable animal for SARS research, but clubbing a civet to death with a metal rod was probably as effective a means of broadcasting the virus as an emergency intubation. In fact, it was a sad testimony that if nobody contracted SARS during the slaughter, the civet probably wasn't to blame for the epidemic.

* * *

After the slaughter, no more cases of community infection emerged, yet at least two questions remained. Did that mean that the civets were, in fact, an animal reservoir for SARS? And did that mean that the live-animal markets of Guangdong were no longer selling civets or other proscribed wildlife? Yuen was of the opinion that the trade had merely gone underground. I decided to see for myself.

I was lucky to have Tan Yue-qiu, a researcher at the University of Hong Kong Institute of Molecular Biology, to take me along, and luckier that he had friends in Shenzhen who were in the restaurant trade, and knew the markets. Don't bring a camera, they warned, or you'll get beaten up.

From downtown Hong Kong to the mainland China border was less than an hour by fast, clean, comfortable train. The border crossing was guarded by the familiar thermal sensors, and the familiar reporting forms were required—and this for one of the busiest border crossings in the world, crossed by nearly half a million people a day.

"We meet my friends," he said, as we crossed a concrete bridge over a trickle eerily like the Tijuana River, along a sidewalk between a railway-terminus-in-progress and a mall, crossed a streetful of manic traffic to a vast, modern hotel outside which we met Tan's friends, Mr. Chen and Mrs. Song, the latter being an old school friend of Tan's wife. They owned three restaurants and a Honda Accord as luxurious as a Lexus. "We go to market first?" Yes.

En route to the market, it became clear that everything I thought I knew about China was wrong. Two decades ago Shenzhen, locally pronounced SnZn, was a fishing village. Now it's like San Diego, but much bigger and less shabby. I'm not usually impressed by big buildings, but so many buildings, so big, so new—it was a little breathtaking.

The market was in a small, scruffy tangle of back streets that must be a relic of the city's fishing-village days. We parked in a police lot whose main feature was a vast statue of a prawn, then headed down a dark, narrow street with small concrete shops on both sides selling the usual cheap plastic market stuff; and there, ahead of us, was the live market, and it was very live, indeed.

Its sides were open; in fact, it seemed to be the open ground floor of a concrete building, perhaps two-thirds the size of a soccer field, supported by concrete pillars. Merchants had set up their wares in rows of cages, tubs, and buckets. In front were tubs of marine life: turtles, frogs, scallops, crabs with their claws bound in twists of leaves, shrimp, crayfish, clawless lobsters, and some enormous kind of clam with a foot like an oxtongue. Just beyond was a low wire cage of live rabbits, with three more cages stacked behind it, full of more rabbits, chickens, and quail.

Inside, the air became thicker with the smell of droppings, or as we now call them, virus fragments. The floor was wet and greasy; it was probably hosed down every so often, but it was impossible to maintain any pretense at sanitation when chickens were excreting on chickens excreting on chickens, in condominiums of contamination. A beggar followed me around as I watched a man skin snakes and toss the flesh in one bucket, the skin in another. The merchants, men and women, many of them with bare feet, glanced in our direction and went back to their cigarettes. The species diversity grew: eel, goats, snakes, small-fry fish of a dozen kinds, ducks, surprisingly docile, like the geese, catfish, cats.

This was fresh, all right—though not uniformly so. Several fish floated belly-up. Four ducks sat on a box, one rubbing the back of its head against the neck of a fifth that had died.

A seller beckoned over our restaurant friends, and lifted a piece of sacking that fell over the front of yet another long, low cage, the top of a stack of four. I couldn't see what was inside, but it was clearly not intended for general viewing. "It is prohibited animal," Tan whispered, but his pocket-calculator-translator couldn't cope, and I never found out what it was.

But if we were in any doubt how shady this place was, we were set straight by a small, white-haired, weatherbeaten man of a certain age who sidled over and told Tan's friends that he could show them wildlife—the key euphemism. It wasn't clear what he had in all, but he certainly had snakes, many of them from endangered species. Not here—back at his house. He would show them to us, but only if we bought and ate some at his place. I'd never been invited to eat an endangered species before. We declined.

Changing practices as deeply embedded in the culture was clearly not going to happen overnight—and later that day we saw how the live markets, far from being an aberration, existed and still exist for good reasons, even if hygiene isn't one of them.

That evening Tan's friends took us a little way up the Pearl River Delta to Yantian Pork, one of a cluster of busy open-front restaurants famous for their seafood, right across the road from the seafront and the fishing boats. The first few yards—the apron—of each of the restaurants consisted of tables, and then there was a row of buckets, a row of large tubs, a row of low tanks, and then three tiers of larger tanks, all filled with seafood. It was simple. You point, we cook.

Again, it was nothing close to hygienic. Nobody wore gloves or hairnets. Someone ahead of me ordered a sole that was scooped out of its tank in a net, tossed into a bucket and put on a scale, whereupon the sole promptly kicked itself out of the bucket and tried to escape across the floor. The server scooped it up and threw it back in the bucket. It was by no means a rough place—in fact, the staff were all friendly, attractive, helpful, well-uniformed—but the customs simply didn't include excessive cleanliness.

I pointed to lobster, sole (not the escapee), oyster, scallop, a kind of bouillabaisse that included turtle and crab, and sea urchin, which you sip, like a custard. The staff asked if I wanted it cooked or raw. Recognizing the limits of my commitment to first-person journalism, I chose cooked. The food arrived swiftly, seasoned and cooked perfectly. It may have been unhygienic, but it was the best seafood I'd ever eaten.

* * *

The cold-and-flu season came and went, and no more SARS cases emerged, though nobody is betting we've seen the last of it.

"I think it will re-emerge," said Dr. Chen Pei-Jer in Taiwan, even before the accident at the CDC lab in Beijing. "The SARS coronavirus is already present in wild animals and in the laboratory, and it will remain a threat unless all the viruses are destroyed, but this is impossible. So if the environment [and the circumstances are] just coincident enough, the virus can cross the barrier and infect humans. However, although this can happen, it will be very hard for it to cause a large outbreak again." It may be like the Ebola virus, he suggested, emerging every few years, "but because we have experience now, we can contain it and reduce its impact."

Chen's research found that the SARS coronavirus mutates relatively slowly, roughly at the rate of polio. This is good news: it means that if and when a vaccine is developed, a single vaccination would probably be good for several years at least. Influenza mutates much more rapidly, and as a result a different vaccine (or bundle of vaccines) is needed each year.

The only other aftershock was not a case at all, but a series of phantom cases: a study discovered SARS antibody in blood samples taken from 17 adults in 2001—before the SARS outbreak. In other words, the virus may have been with us for several years, constantly mutating and adapting but not causing anything especially noticeable in the way of symptoms, and it may have been a single rogue mutation in late 2002, possibly not involving civets at all, that made it deadly.

That unexpected information in particular made it seem as if the SARS outbreak didn't end; it vanished. The whole episode had a curious symmetry, beginning and ending with a few cases in Guangdong, some of them apparently connected to wildlife animals in live markets, and beginning and ending, too, with a cluster of unanswered questions.

By then, chickens were back in the news: an outbreak of avian influenza was running through Southeast Asia and elsewhere, and the morning meetings at Batiment M were reporting on surveillance and containment. A staffer had been hired on a six-month contract to do nothing but file all the emails about SARS, but the members of the Communicable Disease Surveillance and Response Department had other assignments in other countries. David Heymann had been asked to head up the campaign to eradicate polio. The city of Toronto and the province of Ontario were playing brinksmanship over who should pay for public health.

And somewhere in Hong Kong a thin, elderly public employee was standing by an escalator, as people rose in stately procession past him, holding a wad of cotton impregnated with disinfectant against the belt to clean it over and over again.

Chapter 20.

Learning from SARS

When I landed at Hong Kong airport, a year and a day after Professor Liu was admitted to Kwong Wah Hospital, a series of small display monitors above the immigration desks glowed and danced in vivid, abstract designs of greens, whites, and reds. These must be the thermal monitors I'd heard about, I thought. As I wandered toward them in a post-fifteen-hour-flight daze, a slight, pretty, health and immigration officer ran toward me, gesturing: she wanted me to take off my baseball cap so the monitor could register my forehead. Six months after the outbreak, Hong Kong was still on the alert.

By now every major body involved in the SARS outbreak has produced its report, including the lessons to be learned from the experience, and the changes to be recommended. Some of these are universal.

It's clear, for example, that infection control is a weakness everywhere. Health care personnel should be fit-tested for N95 masks before they have to actually use them in an outbreak. Hospitals should have an adequate number of negative-pressure isolation rooms. Bedsheets, coverings, and other equipment that might carry infection should be collected and cleaned or laundered separately. Suitable quarantine plans need to be drawn up before they are needed.

Other lessons are specific to the particular country or institution. A short list of links or references to these can be found in the appendices to this book. Many of them suggest more sweeping reforms in the way public health is funded, the way a nation might protect itself against bioterror, the precautions and planning that might be essential ahead of a pandemic infectious disease other than SARS.

To come up with a catalogue of lessons I personally learned from researching the SARS outbreak may seem self-important and self-indulgent, but I noticed some things that may not be mentioned in those reports, so this is probably the place to say them.

I was struck by how badly all those involved wanted to tell their stories, and how unappreciated they felt; how much harder people will work for others than for themselves, a quality that speaks well for the future of the human race; how much skill and energy, in science and medicine as elsewhere, are wasted on parallel, redundant work, and competition; how spending in health care gravitates toward the wealthy, which means that the wealthy are always going to be terrified of catching the infectious diseases of the poor; and how, strange though it may sound, the countries that had few or no SARS cases missed out on an experience that was devastating but probably of immense value.

Our global ability to react to infectious disease works very much like the human immune system: once we've been infected by some pathogen, our defenses are informed and alert, and we're far better able to suppress the infection next time. The Black Death—the plague epidemic that ravaged Europe in the 14th century—`introduced the importance of quarantine of ships, basic personal hygiene, rodent control, and sewage disposal as central concepts of public health. SARS likewise presents an opportunity for us to be healthier and safer—an opportunity much more likely to be taken seriously by those who had first-hand exposure.

Perhaps the most important lesson, in fact, is that SARS actually happened. It's a peculiar experience to go from Hong Kong, where SARS (and avian influenza) were still very much on everyone's mind, back to the United States, where the outbreak might never have happened, yet where the public is ready to be alarmed by fictional or exaggerated threats every day.

Conventional wisdom in much of the West (apart from Ontario, Canada) has already written off the containment of SARS as a sign that either (a) it was never much of a disease in the first place, or, (b) whatever authorities exist to deal with such problems were and are clearly adequate to the task, and perhaps even that (c) they should have done so more quickly and with less fuss.

"If public health really works well and a health problem is prevented," wrote Barry Bloom in *Science*, "there is little evidence to show that something important was achieved."

This book is part of that evidence.

AFTERWORD

Georges C. Benjamin, M.D., FACP
Executive Director
American Public Health Association

The environment for public health has dramatically changed and public health is much more visible today then ever before. Public health practice is increasingly a "24 hour and 7 day a week" operation in a milieu that demands immediate answers fueled by insatiable media attention. With scientific knowledge advancing at light speed, the pressures on public health practitioners to keep current and effectively use new knowledge remain a significant challenge.

Emerging diseases such as SARS bring new challenges in this changing environment. The potential for explosive spread, the difficulty of regional and international coordination, and the differences in global public health capacity increase the peril. The global nature of the new infectious threats, whether made by man or nature, serves to define a new phase in the history of public health. This phase will either be characterized by the building of a global public health infrastructure to address these risks or defined by the negative outcomes that complacency brings.

The SARS epidemic was initially ignored, then feared, and finally contained. In the countries that took the brunt of the epidemic, SARS was a major public health incident; much like the Anthrax terrorism attacks of 2001 in the United States (U.S.). Over 8,000 people from 29 countries became ill and about 774 died. This is in stark contrast to the approximately 3.8 million people who die annually worldwide from pneumonia, the 2.1 million who die from infectious diarrhea, and the 3.1 million who die from HIV/AIDS.

Put in this perspective, SARS was not “the big one.” It did, however, cost over US$40 billion and served as a global wake–up call. In the end, it was old–fashioned epidemiology and disease control that saved the day: rapid identification of the causative agent, effective communication to the medical care community and the general public, and vigorous disease containment efforts such as hand washing, protective barriers, isolation, and quarantine.

SARS was an excellent exercise in prevention in the United States. Recent preparedness work and infrastructure development after September 11, the 2001 Anthrax attacks, and a dose of luck allowed for an effective U.S. response. The 418 suspected or probable SARS cases with no deaths dispel the myth that the United States was not impacted. Even with no mortality, the amount of time and effort required was massive.

What did we learn?

- U.S. public health infrastructure has improved but is still inadequate.
- A significant sustained investment in resources over a prolonged period of time is necessary to fix the system.
- An accelerated capacity for new basic and applied research to combat new threats is needed.
- Global communication, coordination, and cooperation are essential components for effective preparedness and response.

There is an old saying that when public health does its best work, nothing happens and no one notices. That is still true, but when something does happen, we must be prepared and capable of prompt and effective action.

DIALOGUE

WHO'S David Heymann and Guenael Rodier

At the WHO headquarters in Geneva, David Heymann and Guenael Rodier, frequently finishing each other's sentences and throwing thoughts back and forth across Heymann's desk, identified several lessons from SARS from the WHO's point of view. Rodier spoke accented but technically accomplished English; every so often Heymann would slip into a more informal mode with him, and chat in accented but conversational French like an affectionate older brother, long separated at birth.

Westerners, Rodier started, have developed some genuine respect for their counterparts in Hong Kong, China, and the Philippines. "There are some very good professionals available now in the developing world. When you went to Zaire in the Eighties, you couldn't find many good people, but now you have a lot of good people..."

"With experience," Heymann added, pointing a finger.

"...and good cultural sensitivities, whom we Westerners certainly listen to and admire."

The SARS experience had also shown that outbreaks posed particular difficulties for large decentralized countries such as Canada and, in some respects, China.

"Our relationship is with the federal government," Heymann said, explaining the WHO's charter. "Provincial governments really wanted to share with us preferentially to what they did with their central governments, and that's a non-starter. So the countries have to work on developing a smooth way of working with their provinces and states so the information comes to us through federal government."

"There's no lack of goodwill," Rodier said, "but some countries are very large. It's not that the central governments don't want to share; [it's that] they don't know themselves. In a lot of programs, it takes two, three, four weeks before the minister gets informed."

Questions of communication are closely linked to issues of transparency.

"Because of the enormous economic and political impact of epidemics," Barry Bloom, Dean of the Harvard School of Public Health, wrote in a *Science* editorial entitled "Lessons from SARS," it takes great courage in public health to declare to the world that a country has an epidemic."

This is true, but it may be changing, in two respects. First, news leaks out much more readily with each passing year. Through GPHIN, local media and other unofficial channels, the W.H.O. may well know about an outbreak before the central government does.

"Most of the time now we go to a country to inform them of an event we heard about," Heymann said. "But it's still very important to go to countries for formal verification. It's interesting—in close to two thousand times we've done that, not a single time has a country said, `It's not your business.'"

Rodier looked at an emerging infection from the government's point of view. "It's a natural reaction to want to speak about a problem when you have fully documented it. The problem is that by the time you have fully documented it and reported it, it has leaked out and the whole world is speaking about it!"

The second way in which it may now be somewhat less daunting to accounce to the world that one's country has an epidemic is that sheer pragmatism may be overcoming the stigma and taint of failure.

"When we set out to revise the International Health Regulations (IHR)," Heymann went on, "one of the things we wanted was to destigmatise disease, and make reporting the norm. And I have to say, we've succeeded. People are stumbling over themselves now to report outbreaks of avian influenza. The will to report is now an accepted culture. And if there is an economic [impact], you deal with the economics differently than you deal with the public health threat."

Rodier nodded. "There is no shame. They are concerned about losing money, the business aspect, but there is no shame any more to report an outbreak. HIV in the early 80s to the late 80s it was a shame to report an outbreak. [But now], reporting an outbreak—it's not like a traffic accident, but almost. Speaking freely about an outbreak [now takes place], and it didn't five years ago."

"That's what we strove for," Heymann said. "And SARS gave us the chance."

Each outbreak, in that case, becomes an opportunity for collaboration. Each outbreak also teaches about outbreaks.

"That's another thing," Rodier went on. "We have learned about outbreaks, We don't understand everything, but...we've been collecting different types of outbreaks for the last five years or so. We're starting to have an idea of what is a normal outbreak here. Back to the [analogy of] traffic accidents—what is a normal [occurrence of] traffic accidents? You can predict it—so that, for the U.S. you will have so many accidents a year....

"A baseline." Heymann agreed.

"You have an idea what will happen. We start to have an idea of what will happen globally. You wait for the Ebola season, the cholera season, the influenza season. We need to do moire documentation and analysis, but the professionals start to have an idea of what to expect. Each outbreak is unusual, in a way, but you can spot the ones that are really unusual. Having a huge traffic accident in the middle of the parking lot here at WHO is bizarre, it's not expected. And we start to have the same understanding that a certain kind of outbreak at a certain time in a certain country is..."

"Not expected," said Heymann helpfully.

"Not expected. Today we have a team on Nipah in Bangladesh..."

"But in five years Nipah will be understood. When it occurs, why it occurs...

"...and we have a list of not too many diseases, maybe ten, fifteen diseases that are outbreak-prone, that we start to be familiar with. Still a problem, but we start to be familiar with them."

What other SARS outcomes have they seen?

"The role of the WHO is much better acknowledged," Rodier said. "A lot of countries had respect for the WHO before, but others [less]. But in this area of epidemics, infectious disease, global control and so on I think everyone acknowledges that the WHO has know-how, has something to offer, is the central office in the global system.

"Take the cases of Iraq and SARS, which went on at the same time," Heymann continued. "There was no consensus-building possible on Iraq. With SARS, every country agreed to collaborate. That's incredible. Health has some aspect that peoiple wish to work on. Maybe it's the unknown. I don't know.

"I think there's an understanding that you need all countries to be a little bit disciplined, to follow the same case definition if we're ever to have this common concerted action. Otherwise the epidemic would find a way."

"And the U.S. was not willing to report, at the start, where the cases were coming from," Heymann said, "which was very important for us to know, because it might help identify a new place where cases were coming from. It might say that Canada's [barrier] methods aren't being effective. But we couldn't get that information from the U.S. until quite late in the outbreak."

"Contact tracing is important when it can be done in one country," Rodier explained, "but when it becomes global contact tracing—say someone goes from Hong Kong to Canada to the United States—it requires cooperation between different countries with different cultures. But it worked, more or less, despite that most countries react for themselves. Once they have a case, they say, Never again. They build a wall to protect themselves—but they may not realize that they are themselves playing a role in the international spread. It may not just be you being a victim—you may be a victim and a spreader."

Perhaps the hardest continuing lesson for the WHO is that to some extent every country will and must handle its health issues in its own way. In Hong Kong, for example, it was culturally acceptable to unite the medical and the police databases to help with contact tracing.

"That was not culturally acceptable to Canada," Rodier said. "They also in Hong Kong went into a very detailed rebuilding of the chain of transmission of each and every case and they controlled the outbreak this way. In China it was too big and too difficult [to do that]. They just freeze the country for two weeks..."

"And only China could do that," Heymann put in.

"...And it worked.", Rodier went on. "There are different approaches according to different cultures. In China and Hong Kong the terms in which the outbreak was discussed were military terms, where the highest levels of government were engaged. `We're going to fight SARS,' etcetera. In Canada it was left very much to the public health community. `We have a problem but you're equipped, we're going to hand you the problem.' What I'm trying to say is that from the WHO standpoint you can see the different attitudes."

"In Asia, there was a civic pride", added Heymann. "[And] the attitude was different. In a democracy in Europe or North America maybe we were less equipped when it comes to collective behavior that some Asian cultures or a communist party such as China, [where the government could say] This is the way we're going to do it and we don't discuss it, and if I quarantine you or a quarantine a hundred people there aren't a hundred lawyers popping up and saying, 'You can't do that to my client'."

TIMELINE: SARS

16 November 2002
First known case of SARS is discovered in Guangdong province, China.

January-February 2003
Cases of atypical pneumonia break out all over southern Guangdong province.

11 February
The Chinese Ministry of Health reports that there have been 300 cases including five deaths in Guangdong province from an "acute respiratory syndrome". People in Guandong and Hong Kong start buying vinegar.

17 February
The first SARS case to cross into Hong Kong returns from visiting Henan.

19 February
WHO issues avian flu alert after deaths.

21 February
Professor Liu travels to Hong Kong and checks into the Metropole. Over the next 24 hours or less, at least 16 people staying in or visiting the hotel are infected.

22 February
Professor Liu is admitted to Kwong Wah Hospital.

26 February
First SARS case is admitted to the French Hospital in Hanoi.

1 March
First SARS case is admitted to Tan Tock Seng Hospital in Singapore.

11 March
Health officials realize there is an outbreak of an "acute respiratory syndrome" among workers at the Prince of Wales Hospital in Hong Kong.

13 March
First signs that Toronto may have a SARS outbreak.

15 March
The World Health Organisation (WHO) confirms that Severe Acute Respiratory Syndrome (SARS) is a "worldwide health threat" and that possible cases have been identified in Canada, Indonesia, Philippines, Singapore, Thailand and Vietnam. The WHO issues guidelines warning travellers to South East Asia about the dangers of SARS. A man infected with SARS in Hong Kong flies to Beijing, infecting at least 59 people. A Singapore doctor infected with SARS is removed from a commercial airliner in Frankfurt.

17 March
Virtual lab network established by WHO holds first teleconference to begin identifying the SARS organism.

19 March
SARS spreads to the US and Europe with the UK, Spain, Germany and Slovenia reporting cases.

21 March
SARS coronavirus identified. Official identification announced on April 16.

24 March
Singapore introduces quarantine for probable SARS cases and those who have come in contact with them.

26 March
Cases of SARS begin showing up from Amoy Gardens in Hong Kong.

27 March
WHO recommends screening departing travellers from worst affected areas.

29 March
Dr. Carlo Urbani, the WHO official who first identified SARS, dies of the disease in Bangkok.

2 April
WHO recommends postponement of all non-essential travel to Hong Kong and Guangdong province. Travel to and from most of East and Southeast Asia is dropping precipitously.

5 April
China apologises for its slow response to the SARS outbreak. Several senior officials are fired.

9 April
First SARS case reported in Africa.

14 April
Canadian scientists confirm they have sequenced the genome of the SARS virus.

23 April
WHO recommends postponement of non-essential travel to Toronto, Canada. Travel to and from the city is heavily affected. All schools in Beijing are shut for two weeks in an attempt to halt the spread of the disease.

27 April
Beijing authorities order the closure of all entertainment venues in the Chinese capital—including theatres, cinemas and karaoke bars—until the outbreak is brought under control.

28 April
The WHO says Vietnam has contained the virus, after no new cases are reported in the country for 20 days.

5 May
Chinese authorities quarantine 10,000 people in the eastern city of Nanjing.

15 May
China threatens to execute or jail for life anyone who breaks SARS quarantine orders.

22 May
The infection rate reaches its apex in Taiwan, with 65 new cases in one day.

31 May
The WHO declares Singapore SARS-free.

5 June
The outbreak has peaked around the world—including China—the WHO says.

13 June
The WHO withdraws travel warnings for the Chinese provinces of Hebei, Inner Mongolia, Shanxi and Tianjin, but maintains the warning for Beijing.

17 June
WHO lifts its travel warning for Taiwan.

23 June
China and Hong Kong are removed from the WHO's list of SARS-infected areas.

2 July
Toronto is declared SARS-free by the WHO.

5 July
Taiwan is the last country to be removed from the WHO's list of infected areas.

9 September
Singapore announces that a researcher has SARS, making him the first person to contract the disease in five months.

17 December
Taiwan health officials say a medical researcher at a Taipei military hospital has contracted the virus.

December 2003-January 2004
Four Chinese in Guangdong contract SARS. Against WHO advice, Guangdong officials slaughter an estimated 10,000 civet cats.

ANNOTATED BIBLIOGRAPHY

(a subjective and selective list of further reading)

Web sites:

http://www.sarswatch.org/
No longer being updated, this site is nevertheless a wonderful archive of articles and discussion from a wide variety of sources culled as the outbreak progressed. As such, it's an interesting partner to...

http://www.bikesutra.com/sars/dr_buckley.html
...an archive of email conversations involving Dr. Tom Buckley, a New Zealand physician working at the Prince of Wales Hospital in Hong Kong during the outbreak. Buckley's emails, many of which are exchanges with physicians elsewhere in the world, give a vivid sense of a professional trying to come to grips with an unknown threat in as intelligent and composed a fashion as he can muster.

http://www.hku.hk/sars/index.shtml
http://www.sars.gov.sg/media.html
http://www.taiwantrade.com.tw/TWTRADE/STATIC/sars_0430.htm
http://www.cdc.gov/ncidod/sars/
http://www.who.int/csr/sars/en/
Public-service sites set up by the University of Hong Kong, the government of Singapore, the Taiwan Bureau of Foreign Trade, the U.S. CDC, and the WHO. Most governments and many other institutions established similar pages. It would be interesting to know whether anyone is studying public-service web sites to see

what is most helpful and most effective in terms of content and interactive capability.

http://www.sarsattacks.com/country.php?USA
An archive of blow-by-blow articles about SARS in the United States.

http://www.sciencemag.org/feature/data/sars/index.shtml
A collection of articles, both scholarly and journalistic, about the SARS epidemic. The quality of *Science's* journalism was uniformly high.

Books:

The New Killer Diseases, by Elinor Levy and Mark Fischetti
In our opinion, this book goes along, with Richard Preston's *The Cobra Event* and *The Hot Zone*, as books which can unintentionally induce epidemic hypochondria. Levy and Fischetti introduce some interesting and at times important information, but they do so by following individuals as they meet sad and at times ghastly ends. What they don't show is the hardworking and at times inspired people who stand between us and those diseases, namely...

The Medical Detectives, by Berton Roueche
A delightfully-written series of pieces from the *New Yorker* about epidemiologists and public health employees, who are often as interesting as the process they follow to identify the sources or causes of baffling illnesses, which are often as interesting as the illnesses themselves.

Infections & Inequalities: the modern plagues, by Paul Farmer.
One of the seminal books in social medicine. It does not deal directly with SARS, but its look at how the poorest are disproportionately affected by infectious disease is appropriate context for the SARS outbreak.

Control of Communicable Diseases Manual, 18th edition,
edited by David L. Heymann, MD
A pocket-sized guide, published by the American Public Health Association (which, to disclose fully, also publishes the book you now

hold). It lists all manner of infectious agents and diseases, including SARS, and succinctly describes epidemiology, clinical presentation, methods of control, and medications. It is probably more suited to the physician and public health practitioner than the more lay-oriented...

A Field Guide to Germs, by Wayne Biddle.
An irreverent and selective (yet accurate) version of the above. Humorous, peppered with medical history, and enjoyable whether you do epidemiology and microbiology for a living or just like reading about it.

SARS War: combating the disease, by PC Leung and E. E. Ooi.
It has the distinction of being perhaps the earliest book on SARS. It is somewhat uneven in terms of chapter quality. It is part SARS description, part SARS control manual. One chapter tracks the spread of the disease, another suggests means of control, but nothing quite ties it together—it seems drawn from disparate sources. It is published in Singapore and the authors are from Hong Kong and Singapore respectively—the book is potentially a rich source of local information but somehow short of the mark.

SARS, Governance and the Globalization of Disease,
by David Fidler.
We were kindly provided an advance copy of the manuscript by Prof. Fidler, and much appreciate it. Fidler explains the 'political pathology' of SARS—how the efforts at characterization and control related to the structures of governance and the Westphalian system of international politics. The latter alludes to the creation of modern statehood governance structures. As you can probably tell, not exactly a bedtime page-turner for most people. It is, however, a well-written academic piece, and is worth the effort one puts in to understand the basis for the coordination of SARS control among

different governments and international organizations.
Monographs:

These comprise reports of working groups and expert committees. There are many of these; we list the ones we found most useful.

Learning from SARS: Preparing for the next disease outbreak.
By the Institute of Medicine (IOM), USA.
Somewhat inaccessible for the lay reader, but a trove of SARS-related information from some of the world's leading figures in international health. The book presents chapters based on the presentations and discussions from SARS workshops and round-table discussions. It is an authoritative book on the science of SARS. It has less on the response (since that is an ongoing process), and most of the material herein is current as of October 2003.

SARS in Hong Kong: from experience to action.
Report of The SARS Expert Committee.
This work was commissioned by the Hong Kong Chief Executive, and is similar in scope to the above (the expert committee included Harvey Fineberg, Chair of the US IOM). It focuses particularly on Hong Kong, in terms of the characteristics of the outbreak; issues pertaining to management and administration; and provides specific recommendations for surveillance and control. The lessons learned here would do well to be heeded elsewhere in the world.

Report of the First Meeting of the WHO Scientific Research Advisory Committee on SARS, October 2003.
Similar to the above, but on an international scale.

SARS: status of the outbreak and lessons for the future.
WHO, 20 May 2003.
In contrast to the detailed reports above, this is a concise (10 page) document. One of its more useful features being a timeline with significant events documented.

There are too many articles on SARS to list here; a free on-line search on *Medline* (www.nlm.nih.gov) should provide the latest and greatest. Here are a few we referred to: "The Lessons of SARS." E. J. Emanuel. *Annals of Internal Medicine*, 7 Oct 2003 (Volume 139. No. 7).

Severe Acute Respiratory Syndrome, Beijing, 2003. Wannian Liang, Zongjhan Zhu, Zejun Liu, Xiong He, Weigong Zhou, Daniel Chin, and Anne Schuchat for the SARS Expert Group. Emerging Infectious Diseases (online at www.cdc.gov/eid), January 2004 (Volume 10, No. 1). A very useful reference: The SARS theme issue of *Emerging Infectious Diseases:* February 2004 (Volume 10, No. 2).

ABOUT THE AUTHOR

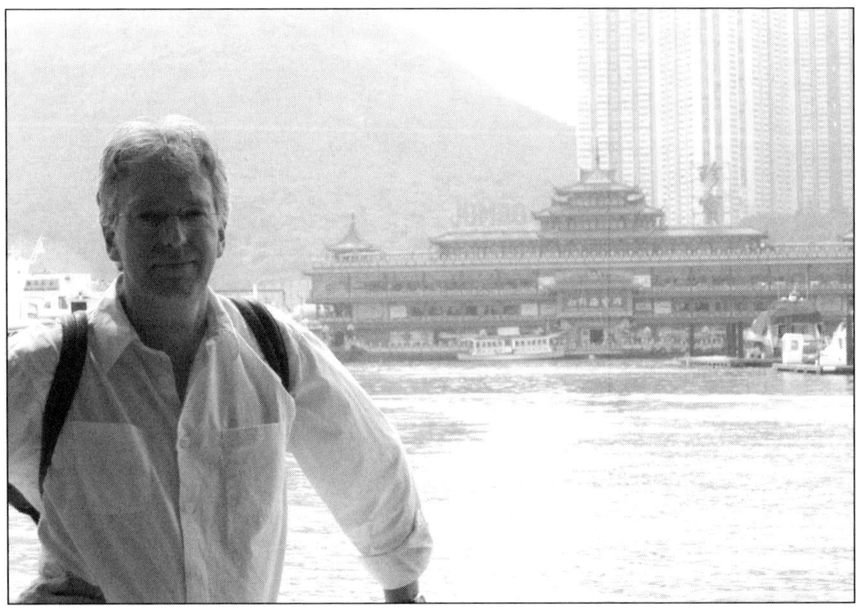

Tim Brookes is the author of books on asthma and hospice care, and is a regular essayist for National Public Radio. He teaches in the professional writing program at Champlain College in Burlington, VT.

INDEX

Academy of Military Medical Sciences' Institute of Microbiology and Epidemiology, China, 102
Adenovirus infection, 29
African trypanosomiasis, 3737
Air purifiers, 54-55
Air travel, 51, 59, 124, 149-159, 181, 192, 205, 219, 221
economic losses from flight cancellations, 155-156
rebound from bans on, 159
to Singapore, 165-168
tourism losses from restrictions on, 155-156
travel bans by individual countries, 154
WHO advisories about, 61-66, 150, 151-159
Alauddin, Sheikh, 171
Amoy Gardens, Hong Kong, 141-147, 153, 188
Ang, Brenda, 75, 91, 186
Anthrax, 29, 35, 109, 218
Antibiotics, 13-14, 54, 86, 102, 109
resistance to, 90
Antibodies to SARS coronavirus, 83, 85, 232
Avian influenza (AI), 4, 232
2002 human cases of, 27-29
first human case of, 5
global alarm about, 33-35
Hong Kong outbreaks from 1998-2002, 7-8
transmission of, 37
WHO alert about, 27, 33
Banlangen granule, 16
Bartlett, Mark, 123-126, 138
Basrur, Sheela, 156
Beijing, China, 15, 28, 193-204
credibility of health authorities in, 203
fever clinics in, 202-203
laboratory transmission of SARS in, 224-225
population exodus from, 198
psychological support for patients in, 200
SARS-designated hospitals in, 200
"unlinked" SARS cases in, 202
WHO office in, 193
Bekedam, Henk, 102, 193-194, 197, 225, 228
Bento, Sherine, 129
Bioterrorism, 218, 225
Blood test for SARS, 82, 111
Bloom, Barry, 119, 234
Bo-Jian, Zheng, 104, 112
British Columbia Cancer Research Center, Vancouver, 115
Bronchiolitis obliterans organizing pneumonia (BOOP), 84
Bronchoscopy, 86, 214
Brudon, Pascale, 47, 48, 50, 151
Brundtland, Gro Harlem, 61, 205
Buckley, Tom, 75

Canada, 52-53, 78, 80, 82, 83, 89-90, 93, 115, 117
airline passenger screening in, 152
cancellations at camps across, 158

Infection Prevention and Control Alliance in, 89
Pandemic Influenza Plan in, 133-134
stigma of SARS in, 187-188, 189, 190
Toronto Public Health efforts in, 121-140
travel advisory in, 153
WHO recommendations regarding travel to, 153, 156-158
Case and Contact Management System (CCMS), 129
Case definition of SARS, 60-63, 80-81
Cell lines, 104, 109, 110-111
Chagas' disease, 36
Chan, Kwok Hung, 110-112
Changjiang, Li, 8
Chee-hwa, Tung, 65
Chi-Leung, Watt, 44-45
Chickens, 1-9, 232
2003 reopening of Hong Kong-China border to, 1, 8-9
deaths in Pearl River Delta, 2-4
H5N1 virus in, 4, 7-8
Infectious Bursal Disease Virus in, 2, 3
slaughtering in Hong Kong, 6-7
Children
impact of school closings in Singapore, 162-164
SARS resistance of, 85
China, 193-204, 226-232
2003 reopening of Hong Kong border to chickens, 1, 8-9
Center for Disease Control and Prevention in, 101-102, 112
decentralized government in, 193-194
domestic travel screening in, 198
downplaying of illness reports in, 15-17, 26
firing of health officials in, 196
food markets and practices in, 229-231
initial SARS cases in, 13-15
initial underreporting of SARS outbreak in, 194-197
public health measures in, 197-201
quality of health care in, 194
quarantine in, 197-198
rumors of illnesses in, 11-13, 16-17
traditional remedies used in, 16-18
travel bans by government of, 154
travel to Hong Kong from, 40
WHO advisory about travel to, 154, 156, 193
Chinese University of Hong Kong, 113-115, 144, 186
Ching, Ken, 95-99
Chiu, Jen-Fu, 142
Chiu, Lily, 76-78
Chiu, Prof., 58
Chlamydial pneumonia, 29, 102-103
Cholera, 21, 35-36, 123, 149
Chrétian, Jean, 190
Chrysanthemum, 18
Chuan, Lee Cheng, 51
Chuanyu, Chen, 12
Chun-wah, Wu, 43
Chunying, Meng, 195
Civet cats, 116, 180, 225-229
Clinton, Bill, 25
Cockroaches, 147, 203
Common cold, 4, 111
Communicable Disease Surveillance and Response Department (CDS), 57, 66
Concert For Toronto, 190
Contact tracing, 41, 83, 97, 153, 213
in China, 194
in Singapore, 166-170
in Toronto, 122, 123, 126-127, 130-132, 215
Containment of SARS, 211, 223, 234
Cooke, Karietha, 130-132, 140, 215
Coronavirus. See SARS coronavirus
Cough, 13, 39, 40, 62, 87, 97, 102
Cunnion, Stephen, 11

Davis, Linda, 121-122
Dengue fever, 37, 51, 82
Diagnosis of SARS, 80-83
by epidemiology, 83, 123

laboratory tests for, 82
sensitivity and specificity of tests for, 82
Diamond, Mark, 158
Diarrhea, 13, 123, 145, 149
Diphtheria, 36
Drug-resistant pathogens, 90
Dubois, Luc, 158
Ducks, 7-8
Duncan, Christopher, 34
Dyer, Gwynne, 33-35

Ebola hemorrhagic fever, 21, 22, 23, 24, 33, 35, 37, 50, 69, 231
Ede, Qin, 102
Emerging infectious diseases, 36
factors associated with spread of, 36-38
global alarm about, 33-35
Global Outbreak Alert and Response Network for, 21-24
modes of transmission of, 36
population growth and, 35
vectors for, 36, 37
End of SARS epidemic, 213, 223, 234
Eng-kiong, Yeoh, 8, 65
England, 186, 189
Epidemic, 1-7
Erasmus University, Rotterdam, 106
Eremita, Alba, 129

Facility-acquired infection, 90, 171, 193
Fever, 13, 39, 40, 53-54, 62, 86, 95, 97, 145
Fischetti, Mark, 90
Food handlers, 14, 226-228
Foot-and-mouth disease, 37
Foshan, China, 2, 12, 13-14
France, 23, 106, 150
French Hospital, Hanoi, 44, 47-50, 73, 149-151
Fu-chun, Margaret Chan Fung, 15
Fujian Province, China, 27-28, 29

Garrett, Laurie, 200
Geese, 7-8
Geographic distribution of SARS cases, 217-218
Gerberding, Julie, 218
Germany, 59-60, 186
Global Influenza Surveillance Network, 28, 48
Global Outbreak Alert and Response Network (GOARN), 21-24, 44, 66-73, 104-105
Global Public Health Intelligence Network (GPHIN), 24-25
Gloving, 91
Goggles, 91
Grein, Tom, 67
Guangdong Province, China, 2, 8-9, 11, 12-15, 28-29, 101-102, 226-228
civet cats in, 226-229
quality of health care in, 194
removal of U.S. State Department employees and families from, 154
WHO advisory about travel to, 154, 193
Guangzhou, China, 2, 11-16, 39
disinfection program in, 16
Respiratory Disease Research Institute in, 102, 195
traditional remedies used in, 16-18
Guangzhou Baiyunshan Pharmaceutical Corporation, 16
Guangzhou Medical University, 44
Gupta, Anuj, 75

Hall, Lyle, 157
Handwashing, 90
Health Canada, 53, 132, 133, 153, 156, 216
Hean, Teo Chee, 163
Henderson, Richard, 186
Heng, Lim Boon, 172
Henry, Bonnie, 82, 83, 118, 122, 125, 129, 133, 134, 136, 140, 164, 176, 214, 215
Hepatitis, 36
Heymann, David, 21-23, 66, 71, 105, 147, 151-153, 158-159, 184, 232
Heymann Doctrine, 21, 71, 105
Heyuan, China, 12, 14

HIV/AIDS, 13, 15, 22, 38, 40, 41, 119
H5N1 virus, 4-5, 7-8., 27-29, 104
Ho, Jimmy, 45, 47, 49-50
Ho Ping Municipal Hospital, Taipei, 207, 209-210
Hohhot Chest Hospital, Inner Mongolia, 195
Hohhot Hospital, Inner Mongolia, 195
Homeless persons, 164
Honeysuckle, 18
Hong, Zhu, 195-196
Hong Kong, 1-9, 39-46
 2003 reopening of China border to chickens, 1, 8-9
 airline passenger screening in, 152
 Amoy Gardens outbreak in, 141-147, 153, 188
 avian influenza outbreaks in, 7-8
 early SARS cases in, 5, 39-40
 expiration of British lease on, 2
 Food and Environmental Hygiene Department of, 146
 influenza epidemics in, 31
 Kwong Wah Hospital in, 43-45, 74-75, 93
 marketplace function of, 2
 Metropole Hotel in, 39-43, 51, 52, 190-191
 Park Lane Hotel in, 95-97
 population geography of, 30-31
 Prince of Wales Hospital in, 51, 53-55, 76, 77, 79, 82, 84-88, 114, 213-214
 Princess Margaret Hospital in, 76-78
 Queen Mary Hospital in, 145
 rumors of illness and paranoia in, 143-145
 slaughtering of chickens in, 6-7
 sporting events in, 170-171, 190
 stigma of SARS in, 188
 travel from China to, 40
 United Christian Hospital in, 91-92, 141
 WHO recommendations regarding travel to, 154, 159
Hong Kong Rugby Sevens, 170-171, 190
Hoping Hospital, Taipei, 182, 193
Hospital for Sick Children, Toronto, 126
Hospitals, 73-93
 French Hospital, Hanoi, 44, 47-50, 73, 149-151
 Ho Ping Municipal Hospital, Taipei, 207, 209-210
 Hohhot Chest Hospital, Inner Mongolia, 195
 Hohhot Hospital, Inner Mongolia, 195
 Hoping Hospital, Taipei, 182, 193
 Hospital for Sick Children, Toronto, 126
 hygiene practices in, 89-91
 infection control measures in, 79, 86-93
 infection control practitioners in, 89
 infection threat in, 73-75, 90
 institutional changes in, 76-79
 Kaohsiung Chang Gung Memorial Hospital, Taiwan, 209
 KK Women's and Children's Hospital, Singapore, 168, 175
 Kwong Wah Hospital, Hong Kong, 43-45, 74-75, 93
 National Taiwan University Hospital, 207
 Prince of Wales Hospital, Hong Kong, 51, 53-55, 76, 77, 79, 82, 84-88, 114, 213-214
 Princess Margaret Hospital, Hong Kong, 76-78
 Queen Mary Hospital, Hong Kong, 145
 SARS diagnosis in, 80-83
 SARS treatment in, 83-85
 Scarborough Grace Hospital, Toronto, 52, 121-122, 215
 Singapore General Hospital, 80, 91, 175, 179
 Sunnybrook Hospital, Toronto, 130
 Tan Tock Seng Hospital, Singapore, 51, 74, 75, 91, 97-

99, 162, 166, 168-171, 182, 186
United Christian Hospital, Hong Kong, 91-92, 141
visitor policies of, 79-80
West Park Hospital, Toronto, 122
Hughes, James, 107, 218-220
Hui, David, 54, 76, 79, 82, 84-88

Identification of SARS coronavirus, 101-113
Infection control measures, 16-19, 86-93, 213-214
for aircraft, 62
in French Hospital, Hanoi, 48-50
in hospitals, 79, 86-93, 122
infection reporting, 19, 41, 43
in Kwong Wah Hospital, Hong Kong, 43-45
N95 masks, 19, 44, 86, 131
negative pressure rooms, 50, 79, 122
personal protective equipment, 91-92, 128, 131
in Prince of Wales Hospital, Hong Kong, 213-214
surgical masks, 16, 17, 40, 54, 86, 129, 131, 142-143
in Tan Tock Seng Hospital, Singapore, 169
in Traditional Chinese Medicine, 16-18
vinegar disinfection, 17-18
Walker Report on, 89
weakness of, 233
WHO recommendations for, 63, 65
Infection control practitioners, 89
Infectious Bursal Disease Virus (IBDV), 2, 3
Influenza Laboratory Network, 25
Influenza vaccine, 25, 38, 95
Influenza viruses, 4, 29, 104, 220-221
Canadian pandemic influenza plan, 133-134
mutation of, 232
U.S. pandemic influenza plan, 221
Inner Mongolia, 51, 195
Institut Pasteur, Paris, 23, 106
Institute for Respiratory Diseases, Guangzhou, 102
International Air Transport Association (IATA), 151, 152
International Health Regulations, 26
Intubation, 84, 88, 92

Jail populations, 164
Japanese encephalitis, 36
Jean-lie, Tseng, 208
Jiabao, Wen, 194, 196, 197
Jianlun, Liu, 39-47, 116
Jiasheng, Chen, 28
Jiaxi, Zhong, 18
Jikai, Li, 196
Jintao, Hu, 196

Kaohsiung Chang Gung Memorial Hospital, Taiwan, 209
Kay-sheung, Paul Chan, 8
Kiang, Lim Hng, 163, 177-178
Kin-wa, Chow, 43
Kindhauser, May Kay, 68
KK Women's and Children's Hospital, Singapore, 168, 175
Kwong Wah Hospital, Hong Kong, 43-45, 74-75, 93

Laboratory tests, 82, 111
Laboratory transmission of SARS, 223-225
Lai-yin, Tse, 15
Lassa fever, 36
Lau, James, 145
Leung, Frederick C., 1-7, 115, 116
Levy, Elinor, 90
Liang cha, 18
Lim, Elaine, 51, 191
Lin, Ruey, 209
Loroza, Nelia, 216
Low, Donald, 83
Lyle, Wendy, 13

Ma-Lin, Ling, 80, 91
Macau, 2, 17, 40
Macintyre, Peter, 128

Mad cow disease, 37, 110
Malaria, 37, 38
Malaysia, 154, 167-168, 180, 181
Manson, Patrick, 31
Mansoor, Osman David, 162
Marburg fever, 37
Mazzulli, Tony, 83
Medecins Sans Frontieres (MSF), 23, 24, 49
Medinfo report, 34
Merianos, Angela, 71, 116
Methicillin-resistant Staphylococcus aureus (MRSA), 90
Metropole Hotel, Hong Kong, 39-43, 51, 52, 190-191
Miranda, Anna, 139
Mok, Ben, 18
Mosquitos, 36-37
  Aedes aegypti, 37
  breeding sites for, 36
  campaigns for control of, 37
Multiple organ system failure, 5
Muscle aches, 13

N95 masks, 19, 44, 86, 91-92, 131, 233
Nanshan, Zhong, 102, 104, 195
National Cancer Centre, Singapore, 179
National Taiwan University Hospital, 207
Nebulizers, 86-88
Negative pressure rooms, 50, 79, 122
Nephew, Geri, 126, 127, 216
Nichol, Angus, 59
Nipah virus, 69

Occupational health surveillance among health care workers, 53-54
Oshitani, Hitoshi, 67, 228
Ostach, Carola, 121-122
Osterhaus, Albert, 106-107
Outbreak, 33, 35

Pak-Leung, Ho, 44
Paramyxovirus, 110
Park Lane Hotel, Hong Kong, 95-97
Pearl River Delta, 2-4, 7, 12
Pei-Jer, Chen, 206, 231
Peiris, Malik, 104, 112
Penfold Park, 7-8
Personal protective equipment, 91-92, 128, 131
Pigs, 4, 6
Plague, 21, 34, 35, 102, 173, 234
Plant, Aileen, 73, 75, 213
Pneumonia, 5, 12, 13-14, 27, 39, 40
  atypical, 13-14, 19
  etiologies of, 29-30
Polymerase chain reaction (PCR), 82, 83, 111
Poon, Leo, 112
Preston, Richard, 35
Prince of Wales Hospital, Hong Kong, 51, 53-55, 76, 77, 79, 82, 84-88, 114, 213-214
Princess Margaret Hospital, Hong Kong, 76-78
ProMED, 24-25, 218
Public health measures
  in China, 197-201
  Global Public Health Intelligence Network, 24-25
  legal issues related to, 135-138
  Toronto Public Health, 121-140

Qi, Huang, 195
Qingdao, Huang, 12
Qingyu, Zhu, 102
Quarantine
  in China, 197-198
  in Singapore, 161
  stigma related to, 187, 191
  in Taiwan, 182-183
  in Toronto, 135-137, 176
Queen Mary Hospital, Hong Kong, 145

Rats, 146-147, 203
Red Cross, 24, 129
Reporting of infections, 19, 41, 63, 121
Reye's syndrome, 5
Ribavirin, 84
Richardson, Karen, 143
Roche Pharmaceutical Company, 17
Rodier, Guenael, 21-23, 66, 71
Rosen, Dan, 70

Ryan, Michael, 22-23, 57-60, 64, 66-72, 204, 222

Salter, Mark, 71, 116
Salvation Army, 129
SARS coronavirus (SARS CoV), 1, 54, 83, 101-119
antibodies to, 83, 85, 232
capricious transmission of, 40, 42
cell lines used in search for, 104, 109, 110-111
civet cat as reservoir for, 116, 225-229
collaborative identification of, 101-113
cross-contamination of West Nile virus samples with, 223
difficulty in obtaining specimens of, 102, 104
future studies of, 119
mutation of, 116, 232
publication of information on, 108-109, 112-113
resistance of children to, 85
sequencing of, 113-116
shedding of, 40, 146
tissue specificity of, 110
vaccine against, 232
virtual network studies of, 116-119
Saudi Arabia, 180
Scarborough Grace Hospital, Toronto, 52, 121-122, 215
School closings in Singapore, 162-163
Schuchat, Anne, 198, 201-203
Scientific journals, 108-109, 113
Scott, Susan, 34
Seiling, Rod, 157
Seng, Alvin, 174
Seng, Chua Hock, 181-182, 192
Sensitivity of diagnostic tests, 82
Sequencing of SARS coronavirus, 113-116
Serum transfusions, 85
Severe Acute Respiratory Syndrome (SARS), 7
capricious transmission of, 40, 42, 118
case definition of, 60-63, 80-81
containment of, 211, 223, 234
diagnosis of, 80-83
early cases of, 5, 39-40
geographic distribution of, 217-218
global awareness of, 48
infection control measures against, 16-19, 86-93
laboratory tests for, 82
laboratory transmission of, 223-225
last cases of, 223-232
lessons learned from, 233-234
naming of, 60, 65
possible causes of, 29, 102-103
resistance of children to, 85
stigma of, 185-195
symptoms of, 13-14, 62-63, 80
treatment of, 83-85
underestimation by physicians, 39, 43, 93
WHO emergency travel advisory about, 61-66
Severe Community-Acquired Pneumonia (SCAP), 19
Shing-jer, Twu, 206, 210
Shui-bian, Chen, 207
Shulman, Les, 131-133
Shyi-kun, Yu, 206
Singapore, 45, 51, 58, 74, 75, 82, 95
Agri-Food and Veterinary Authority in, 180
breaching of quarantine orders in, 176-178, 181-182, 192
end of outbreak in, 183-184
enforcement of quarantine orders in, 174-175, 180-182
Environmental Health Institute of, 223
foreign workers in, 176-177
impact of school closings in, 162-164
KK Women's and Children's Hospital in, 168, 175
Ministry of Health in, 161
National Cancer Centre in, 179
payment for quarantined workers in, 172

public transportation in, 173
quarantine program in, 161-184
Singapore General Hospital in, 80, 91, 175, 179
stigma of SARS in, 186-187, 191-192
Tan Tock Seng Hospital in, 51, 74, 75, 91, 97-99, 162, 166, 168-171, 182, 186
tracking contacts of sick airline passenger arriving in, 165-170
travel from Malaysia to, 167-168
Smallpox, 35, 225
Smyth, Garry, 91, 92, 186
Snow, John, 149
Sore throat, 13, 97, 145
"Spanish flu" pandemic, 5, 34
Specificity of diagnostic tests, 82
Steroids, 84-85
Stigma of SARS, 185-195
Stohr, Klaus, 71, 105-109, 112, 117
Su, Ong Hok, 172
Sunnybrook Hospital, Toronto, 130
Surgical masks, 16, 17, 40, 54, 86, 91, 96-97, 129, 131, 142-143
Swans, 8
Switzer, Barbara, 139, 190
Switzerland, 90, 154
Symptoms of SARS, 13-14, 62-63, 80

Tai, Goh Kee, 161, 170
Taiwan, 51, 182-183, 193, 205-211, 223-224
compensation for medical staff in, 208
Ho Ping Municipal Hospital in, 207, 209-210
initial SARS cases in, 205
Kaohsiung Chang Gung Memorial Hospital in, 209
medical response in, 206-208
nosocomial SARS infections in, 209-210
political responses in, 205-206, 210-211
protests to WHO about status of, 205-206
Tam, Paul, 119, 145
Tamiflu, 17, 83-84, 109
Tan, Gary, 170
Tan Tock Seng Hospital, Singapore, 51, 74, 75, 91, 97-99, 162, 166, 168-171, 182, 186
Tao, Hong, 102-103
Teo, Jolene, 165
Teo, Joseph, 165
Thailand, 150, 155, 219
The Double Helix, 101
The Hot Zone, 33, 35
The New Killer Diseases, 90
Thompson, Dick, 63, 68
To, Ella, 143
Toronto, Canada, 52, 78, 80, 82, 83, 117, 121-140, 232
Bukas-Loob Sa Diyos community in, 187-188
Community Care Access Centre in, 127
Concert For Toronto in, 190
Emergency Medical Services of, 128
exhaustion of health care workers in, 215, 216
lost tourist revenues in, 133
Pandemic Influenza Plan in, 133-134
phase two of epidemic in, 214-216
Scarborough Grace Hospital in, 52, 121-122, 215
stigma of SARS in, 187-188, 189, 190
Sunnybrook Hospital in, 130
West Park Hospital in, 122
WHO recommendations regarding travel to, 153, 156-158
Toronto Public Health (TPH), 121-140, 157, 214
Case and Contact Management System of, 129
case management by, 127
community education by, 138
concerns about SARS in subpopulations, 164
contact tracing by, 122, 123,

126-127, 130-132
containment team of, 130
headquarters of, 124-125
hospital liaisons with, 130-131
information management system of, 128-130
mental health services of, 139
programs suspended during SARS outbreak, 139-140
public health law and, 135-138
quarantine orders issued by, 135-137
recommendations for patient transport, 127-128
reporting by, 133
SARS hotline of, 125, 126
use of Pandemic Influenza Plan by, 133-134
work quarantine program of, 176
Traditional Chinese Medicine, 16-18, 54
Travel advisories of WHO, 61-66, 150, 151-159
Treatment of SARS, 83-85
Tsang, Thomas, 147
Tsui, Stephen, 114, 115
Tuberculosis, 38
multidrug-resistant, 36
Turnbull, David, 156

Umapathi, T., 75
United Christian Hospital, Hong Kong, 91-92, 141
University of Geneva Hospitals, 90
Urbani, Carlo, 47-50, 58, 104, 152
U.S. Centers for Disease Control and Prevention (CDC), 5, 22, 23, 218
Emergency Communications System of, 218
Emergency Operations Center of, 218
Laboratory Response Network of, 220
recommendation for infection control practitioners in hospitals, 89
SARS case definition of, 81
staff deployments to work on SARS, 220
surveillance by Epidemic Information Network of, 218-219

U.S. Department of Defense's Global Emerging Infections Surveillance and Response System (DoD-GEIS), 25
U.S. National Center for Infectious Diseases, 107

Vaccines, 38, 232
influenza, 25, 38, 95
Ventilator dependence, 13-14
Viet Nam, 44, 45, 47-50, 73, 149-151
containment of epidemic in, 213
travel bans by government of, 154
Vinegar, 17-18
Viruses, 2-3
cell lines used in search for, 104, 109, 110-111
coronavirus, 1
H5N1, 4-5, 7-8, 27-29, 104
Infectious Bursal Disease Virus, 2, 3
jumping of species barrier, 4, 7, 36
mutation of, 3-5, 232
relationship to host, 3
SARS coronavirus, 101-119
Vui, Lo Su, 28

Wah-Tak, Kenneth Tsang, 44
Walker Report, 78, 89
Watson, James, 101
Waye, Mary, 113-115, 144-145, 186
Wengkang, Zhang, 194, 196
West Nile virus, 223
West Park Hospital, Toronto, 122
World Health Organization (WHO), 6, 12, 14, 21-26, 42
avian influenza alert of, 27, 33
Beijing office of, 193
Communicable Disease Surveillance and Response Department of, 57, 66
Country Office in Hanoi, 47-48
Geneva headquarters of, 57
Global Influenza Surveillance

Network of, 28, 48
Global Outbreak Alert and
Response Network of, 21-24, 44, 66-73, 104-105
Guide to Hygiene and Sanitation in Aviation by, 62
Influenza Laboratory Network of, 25
initial advisory issued by, 48, 52, 58
mobilizing field teams of, 69-72
outbreak team of, 21-23, 71-72
press office of, 68
requests for help from, 68-69, 157
SARS case definition of, 60-63
situation updates from, 65
travel advisories of, 61-66, 150, 151-159
unprecedented response to SARS outbreak, 63-64, 66-67
Western Pacific Regional Office of, 48, 67, 162
Xenophobia, 96
Xiaoping, Deng, 196
Xuenong, Meng, 196

Yaffe, Barbara, 52-53, 80, 117, 128-129, 214-215
Yang, Annie, 189
Yanga, Nestor, 216
Yanyong, Jiang, 194-195
Yellow fever, 36, 37
Yi, Guan, 104, 112
Ying-jeou, Ma, 208
Yip, Andrew, 43-44, 74, 93
Yue-qiu, Tan, 229
Yuen, Kwok-Yung, 31, 44-45, 103-104, 109-112, 226, 228
Yun, Chen, 196

Zhongshan, China, 2, 12
Zhongshan University, 45
Zhou, Weigong, 203
Zhu, Zhongan, 199-202
Zoonoses, 4, 29, 226